A Man's Cry for Health

A holistic look at a man's mental, physical, &
spiritual health from a woman's perspective

TONI ALIKA HICKMAN

ALIKA PUBLISHING COMPANY
A division of Alikah Enterprise
Houston, Texas

The author of this book recommends methods that are not approved by the FDA. These statements and products have not been evaluated by the FDA. They are not intended to diagnose, treat, cure, or prevent any disease or condition. If you have a health concern or condition, consult a physician. Always consult a trusted health practitioner before modifying your diet, using any new products, drugs, supplements, or doing any new exercises.

I dedicate this book to my sun/son. You are a wonderful spirit & I am so honored you chose me as your mother. I love you beyond infinity. May your strong soul continue to guide you through the obstacles placed in your path, and may the necessary lessons meant to structure your growth come to you with grace, ease, and protection. ~Ase

For my mother, I can never repay you for all that you have done for my sun and I. You are so amazing and such a giver of wisdom and direction. I also love you beyond infinity. Thank you for being a loving grandmother to my sun, and thank you for loving me. You are my ROCK!!

I would like to thank my father, Guy Hickman for allowing me to see that he truly loved me before he transitioned, and trusting me to assist in his transition to the unknown.

I would like to thank all the men who have assisted in my growth as a daughter, mother, a friend, and a lover. Thank you for the joys and pains, the lessons and reflections of my own soul.

For all the men who have been spiritual guides and teachers in my life, I am grateful for your presence and your wisdom that has transcended the male/female boundaries of the human mind concept. Baba Jabade, Brother Danny, Dr.Congo, and all others who have been a part of my journey...I acknowledge you.

To my best friend, Marrio Marshall aka Big Yo. Thank you for believing in me, and thank you for the sincerity of your soul. I truly cherish your energy in my life and appreciate our divine conversations about life and necessary growth. You and your brother did an amazing job on the album/soundtrack to this book, and I hope this project takes our whole team to heights we never imagined so we can continue to create the necessary work we are supposed to give to the world, but on a grander scale! Ase!

Baba Shango- Thank you for being a bright light in my child's life when he needed it the most. He has had the opportunity to have several fathers that have guided his youth to manhood while his biological father has been absent in his life, and you have been a major contribution to his character. I am forever grateful for the time you were in this realm. I/We love you beyond space and time.

Table of Contents

A Man's Cry for Health

Preface

In a world predominantly ran by men, a man's stress levels are elevated by the weight of demand and responsibility expected of him. After birth, many young male children slowly learn about the necessity of mastering their masculinity through receiving beatings and/or verbal punishment from their parents and other adults. If the young male cries he is ridiculed, and grows into an adult who subconsciously understands that he is *not* allowed to show emotion.

Man is truly so much more than strength, hunters, and providers, but because of the UME (united male ego) and the psychological image of mandatory strength that has been placed on his manhood, the importance of health has not been a common discussion for his species. The world is not speaking on health in regards to men, because a lack of health is metaphorically a sign of weakness, and like his tears, society has been trained to look down on his emotional expressions or ailments as weakness.

Because men are so encouraged avoid emotion, they internalize feelings of neglect and depression. According to the Guardian, In the United States, out of 38,000 people who took their own lives in 2010, 79% were men.

This statistic alone show us that men are indeed emotional beings. It also shows us how important it is to get our men to start talking and communicating about their emotions. I remember hearing a quote one time, and it really helped explain the concept of man and woman. "Women are cotton on the outside and steel on the inside, and men are steel on the outside and cotton on the inside." How I digested this quote is; women are emotional beings naturally. We are the nurturers of the world, but are also capable of doing whatever is necessary to provide for our children if need be.

As the women, we MUST be nurturers and emotional beings so we can love our children and the children of the world. We are the mothers of men and the mothers of society. Our intuition and emotions of compassion and empathy when holistically balanced assist us in being a guide for our children and our mate.

However, men are the backbone of our country and our world. They are strong, resilient, beautiful and masculine beings who when holistically balanced, understand that their strength and masculinity is needed to balance our femininity. His cotton is also his extension of his mother and the women who have nurtured this world and his world. Even though ego and male dominated religions have influenced the concept of male/female connection through a woman being born from a man's rib, geneticist have discovered that all human embryos start life as females as well as mammals. I say this only to say that a male's cotton or softer side is not only necessary for his mental, physical, and spiritual balance, but also it is necessary for the male female connection. If he is only steel with no cotton, he is a robot that has no emotion or empathy and controlled by society's programmed thought instead of his own constitution. As a robot, he lacks spirituality and insight. As a holistic completion of man, he is a divine and necessary God energy that channels his life with her life to recreate LIFE. The truth is most of our world, both men and women act as robots, and we both are off balance.

Through television, religion, and social media, we are unconsciously told how to think, act, believe, and even manifest. While I find nothing wrong with having access to all concepts, as human's BE-ing, we have to acknowledge and self-check our ego when it is directing and controlling our thought. We also have to acknowledge when we are allowing too many negative frequencies to influence our spirit.

Though this book is about men's health, it is also about understanding man and helping to define the spiritual and feminine aspects of his nature. As women, we also may need to learn more about the man's body so we can better understand him mentally, physically and spiritually. As his opposite, sometimes we only identify with a man's energy through our emotionally encouraged opinions and often-jaded perspectives. We nurture our young male children the best way we can according to the rules and regulations placed on us from our own childhood. For most of us, we are brought up by our parents with their most sincere intentions of love, but we are also are raised with flaws and generational curses that have been repeated in our family. Some parents have punished and even emasculated our young boys for crying because that is what they have experienced from their own parents. From the bible, to slave masters, to our great grandparents and so on, we have learned that causing our children physical and/or emotional pain is the only way to punish them, and that punishment is the only way.

I know wonderful adults both men and women that were beaten as children and are considered semi-productive citizens of our world. These people encourage causing physical pain to children as a strength, because they believe it is one of the reasons most of society's population consider them successful.

I also know of both men and women who were beaten as a child and they ARE NOT what society considers a productive citizen. The children have still gone to jail, done drugs, and still retaliated in harsh ways just because they finally learned they do not have to be obedient. The young child who received beatings felt pain and fear no matter how they turned out as adults. Both sets of children in this scenario started out as an innocent child, and their perception of life, love, and lack of love ultimately determined how they made decisions growing up.

We all are beautifully flawed,
carrying the challenges of our life
in our soul. ~ Alika Lesson

I have several reasons that encouraged me to write this book. As a Holistic Health Consultant & Naturopath, I was selling herbs and other services, and a male associate wanted to assist me in expanding my product awareness for other men. The concept of only creating a brochure slowly turned into a book. After starting the book, business was picking up and I realized that even though the business was gaining attention, I no longer wanted to do it. An Akashic Reading confirmed my feeling, as my spiritual guides advised me to shut down the herbal site and focus on using my voice, my story, my writing, and my presence on stage to continue my journey in healing.

I grew up in a single mother household, with summer time visits to my father in Atlanta. My trips to Atlanta stopped when I was 10 years old, because my father's new wife decided she did not want me in her house anymore. In turn, I grew up with daddy issues. After I became an adult, my dad and I made peace, but it was a long road of anger and abandonment energies that I held in my soul. Yet, even though I made peace with my father before he transitioned, I realized that my faith in men was depleted because my father rejected me when I needed him. Some people say, "Oh, you just have to get over it," but how do you get over it if you never have that conversation? Well, you never get over it.

The memory will never leave in regards to the pains that are placed on a child forced to live without another parent for whatever that reason may be. I have many men in my life now that I have adopted throughout my lifetime. One of my best friends is a man who I have had several conversations with about understanding the male-female relationship. It is through all of my relationships with men, including my only male child, my light, my sun, that I have discovered how important it is for women to have a deeper understanding of the male species.

Another reason I decided to write this book is because I have male clients who do not have health insurance, and through consultation, I have learned the frustrations and challenges men go through with their health issues.

Even though it is known that women will neglect their own health to take care of their family, the world focuses more on women's health than men's health. 52% of men suffer from erectile dysfunction, 1 in 7 men will suffer from prostate cancer in their lifetime, 1 in 8 men are diagnosed with depression or some other form of mental illness and heart disease is the leading cause of death for men with 1 out of every 4 deaths being heart disease. Most men die at a faster rate than women do, and yet the majority of society still focuses on the woman, her weakness, her health or lack of, and her beauty or lack of.

"The commercial attention on the adult male character is identified mostly by money, dominance, sex and power."~Alika Lesson

My hope is that my book, "A Man's Cry for Health," will spark conversation about the majority of questions men have concerning their own physical health, while also stimulating ideas on his mental and spiritual health. I also hope that the women and mothers of our world can gain insight from the information provided, so we may be better mates, nurturers, and healers to our men. I have included interviews from a few different men and I hope that it brings up ideas and conclusions for all of us. As I write any of my books I asked that spirit guide me during the entire process so I may be of service to all who chose to read. I ask that spirit guide me to give the reader the right information, right thought, and right guidance toward the elevation of a higher knowledge of self. I love you. ~Ase

A Man's Cry for Health

A Man's Cry for Health- Song

They say you got a chip on ya shoulder/
More like a bolder/
In your back like that with the weight of the world
and it just gets colder/
He on that lean, he on that Ex/
He smoking weed, he thinking sex/
Whole world gone mad and his soul is so sad/
So I try and help you ease the pain..

You know I hate to see you cry
Baby I
Hate to see you cry

I hate to see you cry
Eye eye eye eye eye eye
I hate to see you cry
Eye eye eye eye eye eye

Activate
You know I hate to see you so frustrated
I know sometimes your life is complicated
You questioning if life is overrated
It's not my baby
Life is amazing
And you're amazing
God in the flesh
I got ya back
Lay on my breast
When you feel attacked
By this cold world
'cause every strong man really needs a strong girl

A Man's Cry for Health

And I am here for you
What you need bae
Just tell me what you need bae
Tell me what I need to do
To save your soul

They say you got a chip on ya shoulder/
More like a bolder/
In your back like that with the weight of the world
and it just gets colder/
He on that lean, he on that Ex/
He smoking weed, he thinking sex/
Whole world gone mad and his soul is so sad/
So I try and help you ease the pain..

You know I hate to see you cry
Baby I
Hate to see you cry

A Man's Cry for Health

Get the Album at www.tonihickman.com

I Believe in You

As human's BE-ing in today's world, we are able to celebrate our victories as well as have instant ego gratification through social media and other online sources via the internet. Unfortunately, the destruction of the human BE-ing is also instantly advertised for the whole world to see, thus promoting a demeaned reflection of a person's character and shattering confidence that has been built over a period of time.

Believing in yourself and maintaining confidence can be a challenge when we live in a capitalistic society that thrives on the foundation of monetary advancement as the prime image for success.

> *"Although money is definitely a key to building a successful foundation, the integrity of the soul shouldn't be compromised by materialistic gains that are purchased for egotistical gratification."~Alika Lesson*

So many of us end up working jobs that we hate and repeating a cycle of negligence to our spirit because while we acknowledge that we are spiritually unhappy at our job, we still continue to emotionally suffer for the sake of financial stability. The truth is you are never required to do a job that makes you cringe every time you go to work. When we feel anxiety and regret consistently in the soul, that feeling is your soul speaking to you saying, "This is not a good choice."

Now don't get me wrong, jobs teach us lessons we need in life, whether we OWN them or not. Jobs teach us about public relations, responsibility, sacrifice, flawed character in other humans, as well as ourselves. It is when we choose to receive the lesson; a job is the best teacher of the trials and errors of business.

"We all have gifts we are born with that we must give back to the world. We have to develop our gift so it makes the world a better place, and when our gifts are truly developed, our gift will take care of us."
~Danny Russo

What Brother Danny is saying is that our gifts/talents that we are born with are also our financial stability when we decide to use our gift it in its God Bodied form.

For me, my gift has always been anything to do with stage and the creative arts. In church, I remember taking the microphone from a young man standing next to me, because it was my turn to sing and he was taking his time giving me the microphone. I wanted to sing and perform at that very moment! From there I went on to performing in talent shows, singing, rapping, dancing, and doing motivational speaking. I eventually signed to a major record label and featured on gold & platinum albums.

Our gifts vary from each individual. Your gift may be a curious mind that eventually ends up creating the first teleport machine that transcends space and time. Alternatively, you may be the first person to build train transportation in the sky. The key to finding your gift is the same key that opens a passionate joy in your heart when you participate in doing that particular activity.

Whatever your dreams are, whether you are young or old, I hope you will live them. I hope you will acknowledge your purpose and share your purpose with the world, and not allow fear and negative thinking to take control of your magnificent brain. If you are a replica of God's image, this means that you too have the capabilities of being a God..Actually, you are a god, and you alone have the power to change your reality.

I just want you to know that no matter what expectations the world puts on you, I really do believe in your magnificence. If you are ever feeling lost and discouraged, remind yourself that all is temporary and pain usually comes with the gift of lesson. Greed, Envy, Lust, Pride, Laziness, Anger, & Gluttony are the seven deadly sins according to the bible. They are also the many reasons we end up suffering and in low vibrational situations. It is so important to be obedient to our inner soul, because the inner voice is the voice of God/Your Higher Self guiding you to correction. When we are obedient to our souls/God/Higher Self, we have the ability to be amazing.

Therefore, no matter what sin/low-vibrational choice you make, you will eventually suffer because of it. However, if we decide to make good choices for our life, we will reap the benefits of good choices. Simple right? You are capable of making positive choices for your life. You don't have to live a life of extreme suffering, depression, drugs and death.

"We must give up the silly idea of folding our hands and waiting on God to do everything for us. If God had intended for that, he would not have given us a mind. Whatever you want in life, you must make up your mind to do it for yourself."~Marcus Garvey

"Ye Are Gods; and all of you are children of the most high." ~Psalm 82:6

What Is A Phallus?

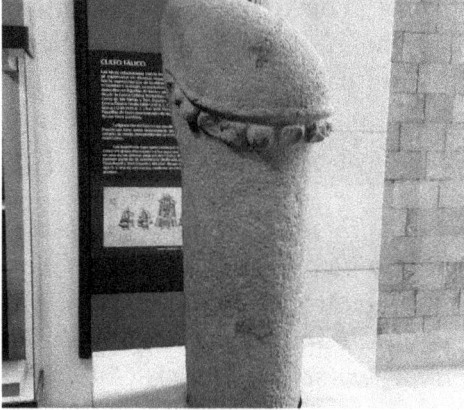

Image taken in Mexico City's Mayan Museum.

I had the opportunity to travel to a few cities in Mexico in 2016. While we were visiting, I was able to climb the Teotihuacan pyramid, visit Chichen Itza pyramids, and visit Mexico City's Mayan Museum. It is in the Mayan museum that I took a picture of the Phallus. When I first saw it, I was a little shocked, as it was so big and erect! I was not sexually fanaticizing about the gigantic penis, but it really spoke for the potential of man's nature. I later discovered that several countries throughout the world worship the penis and host Phallus festivals.

When I first moved to Houston, Texas, from Atlanta, Georgia, I became fascinated with Egyptian/Kemet History. This was actually the first time I was taught about the phallus. According to some Kemet stories, Set killed Ausar (Osiris). Now, Ausar was the God of the dead in some stories, and some he was the Kemet (Egyptian) God of vegetation and civilization, other stories he is simply referred to as God. He was one of the children of Geb and Nut, and married to his sister (Auset) Isis and they were twins. Ausar (Osiris) represented the male productive force in nature, while Isis was the female productive force in nature.

Osiris was murdered by his evil brother Seth, who also tore his body to 14 pieces that were thrown in the Nile (Some stories say he was nailed in a coffin and sent down the Nile River, where Set then scattered his body throughout Kemet). However, Isis found and embalmed his scattered remains with the help of the god Anpu (Anubis). She used magic to resurrect Osiris. Osiris's phallus/penis was turned into gold, (Some stories say the magic was done by Isis, and some say by Anpu) it is with this magic Phallus that she was able to give birth to her son/sun, Heru.

Once Isis knew she was pregnant with Heru/Horus, she fled to the Nile Delta marshlands to hide from her brother Seth who jealously killed Osiris and who she knew would want to kill their son. It was in the Nile that Isis birthed a divine son, Heru (Horus).

The Phallus Obsession

The obsession with the male penis has been developing sent B.C. (before Christ). The story of Ausar, Auset, and Heru is actually an earlier version of the holy Trinity in the Bible. With that being said, one can certainly understand the obsession of the phallus (penis) and its power. Subconsciously, the penis is connected to magic, life, and superior strength. After all, it is the Golden phallus that created Heru (Jesus), and when Seth tried to kill him, he was resurrected in three days.

Technically, the penis is not supposed to die. It is the human/spirit life force, which is why men can continue to make babies long after their female counterparts have gone through menopause (menopause is debatable, I know..Another time). This is also why so many companies cater to the male erection, but ignore his spiritual essence. The world of commerce promotes sexual thought through pornography, commercials, strip clubs, music videos, and more to arouse man's sexual thinking.

It was in my psychology class that I learned how frequently the majority of men think about sex. According to my male psychology professor, the average man thinks about sex every 17 seconds. When I researched the numbers, some statistics say he thinks about sex more than 17 seconds, and some say less, but the average is 17 seconds in America. As women, we know that men think about sex often, which is one of the reasons many of us dress in fashion that appeals to his wandering eye. It is one of our ways of intentionally activating the pheromones.

Most women really enjoy sex with our male counterparts if we are not gay, or if we do not have the psychological issues that come with being raped or abused. However, our womb & Isis energy connects the majority of us to a nurturing spirit, and nurturing energy is connected to the heart. Therefore, although we enjoy getting our freak on, it is our nature to have loving and nurturing feelings for our mate. Even when women say they just want sex from a stranger, they are either fulfilling a lack of love that has come from men, or choosing to go against our divine nature (I have definitely done this). Many times as women, our desire for an emotional connection has caused us to fail in sexual relationships and spiritually intimate relationships, because we failed in seeing that sex and spirituality are not separate. When we (male and female) decided to take the spiritual part out of sex, we denied ourselves of sexual evolution.

Truthpaste-*I have only had one spiritually sexual experience in my life.*

17

Phallic Architecture

Phallic architecture consciously or unconsciously creates a symbolic representation of the phallus. Buildings intentionally or unintentionally resembling the human penis are a source of amusement to locals and tourists in various places around the world. Also, most Christian and catholic buildings, as well as state capitol buildings in the United States are a resemblance of the Male Phallus.

Buildings and Structures that are Phallus inspired

Empire State Building
Leaning Tower of Pisa
Nelson's Column
Colonna Mediterranean
Obelisk of Luxor
Oriental Pearl TV Tower
State Capitol, Lincoln
Torre Agbar
Washington Monument
Christian Science Church, Dixon, Ill
Hyde Park, Hyde, Greater Manchester
People's Daily Tower
Hyde Park Obelisk, Sydney

A Mother & Her Sun

When I gave birth to my only child, I must say that he was a much-needed bright light in my life. Around the time my sun/son was born, I was going through some difficulties with his father, as well as postpartum depression. I went from being a music artist that was working with heavy hitters in the music industry to falling in love with a man that spoiled me rotten, and eventually I became *just* his "Baby Mama." The more my sun's father & I grew, the more I just let him take care of me. I stopped doing my music, I didn't work, and my only responsibility was making sure I kept the condominium clean that he was renting for me and cooked. I gave my power away..Not because he asked me to, but because I thought I should be willing to do anything to make sure the love I had for him was always available. I liked the illusion of being a KEPT woman and leaving all the financial responsibilities on him. I was so lost in being in love and trying to make sure the love would never leave that I could not see how I was isolating myself from my own purpose, nor how my delusional mentality made me needy and weak. I later learned that giving my power away was the wrong choice for several reasons, and it is a choice I will never make again.

Becoming a mother was the beginning of me fulfilling purpose. No matter what my sun's father and I went through, when I would see my sun's face while breast-feeding, or changing his diaper, or simply just holding him, it would make my heart melt. I slowly realized that I was going to be responsible for this young male's growth, and he would have to grow up absent of a father. As I have been able to watch him grow, I have experienced his pains and reactions to a sometimes -harsh world. Being a mother to a young melanin dominant male, we see first hand what the male needs, how he changes, and how the world is afraid of him if he doesn't look like a well-groomed (according to planted thought expectation) man. Watching him rejected by other melanin dominant groups can also be disturbing to his own understanding of who he is supposed to be.

My sun is the first child of our family that was not indoctrinated by religion and its belief systems. Even though he has a fair understanding of church because he has been to church with different friends in his life, I wanted him to develop his own perception about who God was in his life, while also understanding that God/Source is his highest form of energy that operates in mostly all of us. He has partially been homeschooled by me, but I was not the best teacher during this time because I was also a single mother trying to manage the bills and balance the challenges of what two brain aneurysms & a stroke did to some of my thought processing. So then magically, my sun won a scholarship to an African centered private school where he learned not only about the amazing melanin dominant leaders that our children are never taught about in the public school system, but he also learned about the different spiritual systems that were used before man created religion. He eventually went back to a charter school, but he went with a greater knowledge of self.

I do not think I have been the world's greatest mother by any means, but it was important for me to make sure that my sun was not trained to believe he could only think one way about his spirituality. I also wanted to make sure that he knew God lived inside of him and he always holds the power to change his own reality. When he comes to me and says, "I don't feel right." I ask, "In your spirit or do you feel sick?" He will respond with either, "My stomach or head hurts," or "I'm getting some bad energy from someone," or simply "I feel bad in my spirit."

Spirit Talk: When we allow our children to maintain their own sense of wonder and not tell/train them how to think, we allow their minds to develop their own beliefs and concepts about life and spirituality. No matter what religion it is, all of them have a common thread, the Buddhist call it The Noble Eightfold Path.

The Noble Eightfold Path Summary

- ***Right understanding.***
- ***Right thought.***
- ***Right speech***
- ***Right conduct.***
- ***Right means of making a living.***
- ***Right mental attitude or effort.***
- ***Right mindfulness***
- ***Right concentration***

The best thing we can do for our children is to cater to their soul development just as much as we cater to their potential for material success. Teaching them to listen to their spirit will guide them in their decision making process when they are faced with choices that require the spiritual advice of intuition.

A Man's Hair

I remember a time when I was hosting & promoting an event in Houston, Texas. I ran into the president of a certain established mentoring group at a park close to Texas Southern University. The group, to whom I will not mention their name, were known for being mentors to melanin dominant males, & I was so excited about the possibility of getting my sun into their program. My sun & I walked up to the president of this organization and started inquiring about the ongoing mentorship program. When I asked about the process of entering my young king into the program, he immediately looked at my sun and said, "He would have to cut his hair before we even consider him." My sun looked at me, and then looked at him and politely said, "I am not cutting my hair."

We grow up with perceptions of thoughts planted into our psyche. Mainly humans have taught us how to think, what to wear, who is beautiful, what to believe about God, Who is acceptable, what the color of your skin means, etc. We then take what we have learned and unconsciously embrace it as part of our behavior. Then, we place our *taught* thought about what we believe should be, on other humans and we end up operating under taught thought instead of trusting our intuition. When melanin dominant people were captured, one of the first things the slave owners would do is cut our hair to take away our sense of identity. Now, we as a people who have overcome so many hardships have accepted that our hair/skin/culture needs to be altered in order to succeed.

At first, I was deeply disappointed in the leader of this group for wanting to put my sun in an either/or situation. Then, I simply realized that I needed to make sure he was never in *any* group that wanted to alter his naturally kinky hair for acceptance or make him feel less than because he has hair like (wool) Jesus.. Now, if cutting my sun's hair was something that my sun wanted to do because he just wanted to change his look, I will support it 100 percent! However, as melanin dominant people that are born with naturally coiled hair, we have also been trained to think that our hair and our skin is a problem. We have been taught that society will accept us if we adapt to the image *they* would prefer to see on a melanin dominant person. I wanted to make sure that I taught my sun his truth about his culture. I wanted him to know that his ancestors were kings and queens, and that because his dad was Nigerian, his blood and deep melanin colored skin was proof that his blood is rich and he is a true child of royal blood.

Unfortunately, we do live in a world where melanin dominant people are judged by our hair, so the easier choice to get along with society is to cut for men, or perm for women. For the record, I have no problem with whatever choice a person makes for their hair if they are not influenced by the stigmas of society. We have been cutting, shaving, wearing weaves and wigs since before slavery existed, so this too is a part of our culture. However, if your choice to shave your head is because you care about what other races and other melanin dominant people will think with their tainted perceptions, I ask you to do some soul searching. We have the power within us to change the expectations of natural hair in the media, but first we have to believe in our own image of self.

There is rumor of an experiment done on a group of male Indians during the times of the Vietnam War. The government decided to pull the most powerful Indian men, who were known in their tribe to be strong, alert, and highly intuitive. These men also had long hair and beards. During the experiment, the powers that be would have these men do testing that required their intuition, such as having other soldiers sneak up on them, or/and setting traps for them etc. The men scored high when they had all of their hair intact. However, when the hair of these same men was shaved, the men failed horribly. The conclusion of this study was that the men were more intuitive & alert when they had hair.

On another note, Many Egyptians started shaving because they thought our hair was viewed as a symbol of a man's animalistic energy.

Then, there is the story of Samson and Delilah. Samson was known for his strength as a warrior that came from his uncut hair. When Delilah had his seven locs shaved, it weakened him and the Philistines seized him and took out his eyes…hmmm. Metaphorically, one has to see the hair/eye connection of this story. When we cannot see with our eyes, we rely on our intuition to guide us. Without his hair and his eyes, he was completely lost.

The hair acts like antennas for the soul. It allows us to tune in to the universe with better reception. This is why when we get scared, or have a shocking emotional reaction, the hairs on our arms literally "Stand up."

Absent Fathers

I am one of many women who have experienced an absent father in the household. Fathers.com says, "More than 20 million children live in a home without the physical presence of a father. Millions more have dads who are physically present, but emotionally absent.

"If it were classified as a disease, fatherlessness would be an epidemic worthy of attention as a national emergency." ~National Center for Fathering

I actually grew up in a fatherless household. This situation eventually gave me "Daddy Issues," and I saw that my relationships with men were tainted because my father pushed me away for another woman. Therefore, in return, I would either push the men away that wanted to date me because psychologically if I allowed myself to get close they would have the power to hurt me like my own father did. However, if I did not manage to push him away, I ended up being too clingy and loosing myself in thought about him instead of my own progression. The love and pain that I have gone through in dealing with my sun's father really helped me balance *some* of my Father issues, and the pain I experienced with my 2 brain aneurysms and stroke reminded me of how important it was for me to fall in love with myself. I was able to forgive my father before he transitioned, and assist him in his journey to the next realm. In addition, even though I held lots of anger towards my child's father in the beginning of my sun's life, I have also forgiven my sun's father.

Lesson from Spirit

I have learned that I cannot be responsible for carrying any emotions about other people's choices. If I have to be honest with myself, then I have to admit that some of my actions and choices in regards to my sun's father were not from spirit, but from ego as well. Carrying anger around because of another person's choice is unhealthy for the heart and the soul. As the old spiritual saying goes, in many situations we have to learn to, "Let go and let God/Spirit/ Higher Self/ Source."

We all have the power to make better choices for the greater good of our world. Even though society made it easy to paint the picture of Melanin Dominant men not being around for their children, my eyes have been able to witness the magnificence of fatherhood throughout the Melanin Dominant community. A message for those fathers who are not currently in your child's life and still have an opportunity to make a better choice: He/She needs the highest part of you to be a guide in shaping their perceptions on receiving love from a divine male energy.

Understanding that some fathers may never return, or have had an unplanned transition out of this realm, we single mothers have the opportunity to build our child's character the best we can, while also trusting that what we are not able to provide as mothers, will be provided by lessons and people sent directly from God/Spirit/Higher self/Source. We have to know that our child is protected at all times by the most high, and we have to let go of the anger if we carry it towards our "Baby Daddy," and acknowledge that we were able to bring a life into this world because of him. If he returns with sincere intention towards being a father to his seed, we must allow regardless of our personal issues with him if he has not crossed the line. People make mistakes. Some people learn from mistakes, some people do not.

On a final note, if the father never comes back in his child's life by choice, then maybe their presence would have done more harm than good towards the development of your/our child's destiny. I am learning that some things may look like bad things, but are actually good things. In addition, sometimes we just do not have the answers and have to trust that all is divine. In this moment, our child is still a reflection of God/Spirit/Higher Self/ Source. ~Ase (and so it is)

God is Both Man & Woman

Ha! Ha! This is not a debate!

The reality is all babies are female in the womb until they reach a certain peak. According to men's health, "Everyone comes from a common genetic and developmental framework that is tweaked by sex hormones," says Richard Bribiescas, Ph.D., director of the Yale Reproductive Ecology Laboratory. "We all start as a generic embryo. You have a set of male or female sex chromosomes, but the distinction doesn't kick in until your hormones enter the picture," he explains. "Without hormones like testosterone, you would stay on the path to womanhood. And, sorry to say, your body already started developing by the time this decision was made—which means your lady parts were already starting to form."

This does not mean man was born to be gay or transgender, this means that we all have a masculine and a feminine side. This fact also supports the theory that woman is God, but that is another story. The problem is that the united subconscious of thought has deemed woman as weak and fragile, which in turn influences man to not want to identify with his feminine side because by society's standards, man's identity of strength is absent of female energy.

A Man's Cry for Health

The life of a man is so much more than physical strength and erections. In a healthy state, he is a high vibration of love, protection and honor. He is a warrior and provider for his family, a father, and a great mate. He honors his body and eats a healthy diet. When he is in a healthy state, he is erect in his spirit and he is a giver of positive energy, discipline, and strength. In an unhealthy state, he is a low vibration of abuse with himself via drugs, people and circumstances, which holds a potential for manipulation. He does not respect himself or those around him. He eats low vibration food like products, and for the right amount of material possessions, he has no loyalty or honor. The low vibration man has insecurities and allows his ego to overpower his reasoning. The same applies to the low vibrational woman.

What I have learned in my years living in this realm is that we all can fluctuate between a high and low vibration of self. Even the most spiritually grounded human has a shadow self that they can only suppress for so long before those thoughts of negative action and or negative thought surface. At times, we all can lack compassion and empathy towards our fellow human being if their current situation doesn't fit our idealized perception of who and what we thing they should be. For myself I am learning to embrace the shadow part of me so I can grow to my fullest potential. You see, good or bad, right or wrong and all other opposites actually separate us from ourselves. It is from our bad experiences that we learn our path. Therefore, just because a man is operating from a low vibration does not mean that current person is whom he will forever be. Man is forever becoming and growing into the unknown. Even in his weakest moments, he is discovering the power of his strength.

Adding Spiritual Intimacy

Before I started this chapter, I prayed to the energies that work with my soul so I can deliver this message without ego and my biased opinion.

As a woman, it is easy to think all men are controlled by the head of their penis, however, I have been able to meet some awesome men (very few) who have mastered control of their animalistic self.

I fully acknowledge that one of man's divine purposes on this earth is to procreate. I also acknowledge that men are programmed by Mother Nature herself to seek women first for the sake of planting the seed of life in her body and procreation. Yet, men also enjoy sex because they like the feeling of inserting their penis into a woman's vagina. Many spiritual teachers have explained the woman's vagina as a spiritual gateway, while some teachers have even called the woman's womb, heaven. They have also described the man's penis/phallus as a portal of life. The womb of a woman is the nest for a human/spiritual life force to reincarnate, and is literally responsible for carrying and nurturing another spirit. On the other hand, the male has a sacred responsibility to be the vessel in which life is rocketed off into the womb through his penis for a spiritual manifestation. Both male and female sperm are responsible for creating life, but sex is mandatory for the concussive force between both energies to manifest another living being.

In this regard, sex is the most spiritual experience we can ever encounter because we are literally connecting with another soul through intimacy. Unfortunately, my pastor never taught me that sex was a spiritual experience. Many of us have grown up with guilt and shame because we have not been properly educated about sex on a spiritual level.

I started reading books on Tantra about five years ago. I was fascinated by the concept of adding spirituality to intimacy! When I started reading these books, I was also going through my 6 years of celibacy and working on healing the spiritual and emotional pains of my own womb, so the thought of combining my renewed yoni energy with someone of complimentary vibes was literally filling my imagination with wonderful thoughts.

As I write this book, I am also admitting that I have only had one spiritually sexual experience. I say this because my channeling messages for this book comes from spirit, but my flesh has only began to learn about the art of discipline and release required between the male/female energy to achieve fulfillment in Tantra and channeling the kundalini.

Spiritual intimacy takes effort, mediation, and a divine and trusting feeling of openness. I have by no means mastered the art of spiritual intimacy, but what I am learning is that spiritual intimacy is truly freedom, and a path that my partner must be open to bring into our relationship.

Rev. Shawn Wells Goldman is a shaman that is featured in the back of my book. His wife is an Oracle, and I have personally witnessed their truths that come forth through sex magic. There is absolutely no way she would have had access to the information I requested of her before she was able to enter the spirit realm through sexual intimacy with her mate. She also teaches on this subject, so please visit her site at bthevibe.com.

I will also list recommended books in the back of this book for those interested in diving deeper into the sacred sex topics.

The following information may be a subject that we learned in school, but this book is a reminder of what we tend to forget after our educated forced learning sessions are over. It is also a way to look at the lesson from a different perspective. I hope this information provided will assist in the relearning about the male body as much as possible. I believe the more we know about how our bodies function, the more we will know when something is, "Off."

Male Reproductive System

The male reproductive system, like that of the female, consists of those organs whose function is to produce a new individual, i.e., to accomplish reproduction. This system consists of a pair of testes and a network of excretory ducts (epididymis, ductus deferens (vas deferens), and ejaculatory ducts), seminal vesicles, the prostate, the bulbourethral glands, and the penis.

Male Reproductive System

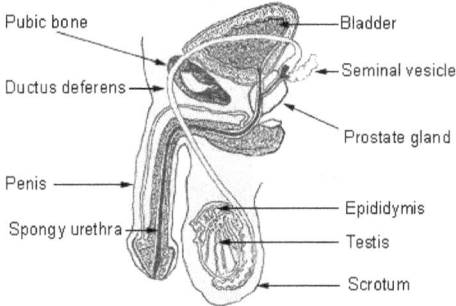

Inside and outside
- The testes (balls) are where sperm is produced and stored once a boy has entered puberty. The testes are also the body's main source of male hormones.
- The scrotum is the sac of skin which holds the testes in place outside the body.
- The prostate gland is located near the bladder and is involved in urination as well as ejaculation. It produces fluid which forms part of semen.

- The vas deferens is a tube that carries the sperm from the testes to the urethra.
- The penis is an external male sex organ through which semen passes during sex. The penis is also used for urination. Penises come in different shapes, colors and sizes.
- The foreskin is a fold of skin that covers the top of the penis. Sometimes the foreskin is removed surgically at birth in a procedure known as circumcision. The penis works the same way whether or not it has a foreskin.

The testes

During puberty, your testicles (testes) change and begin to produce the male hormone testosterone and sperm. Sperm are tadpole shaped and their 'tails' help them move. Sperm are so tiny that they can only be seen under a microscope.

Testicles need to stay cool for sperm to develop normally. This is why they hang outside the body in a sac (bag/balls) called the scrotum. It is quite normal for one testicle to be larger or to hang lower than the other.

The penis
Penises vary in size and appearance. The sizes of adult penises vary, but when they are erect (hard), they are mostly a similar size. When the penis is stimulated or a guy is sexually aroused, the penis can grow from being small, limp and soft to larger, erect and hard. This is called an erection. The penis does not contain any bones and is not made of muscle. The penis becomes erect because the tissue inside the penis fills with blood under pressure.

The foreskin is a fold of skin which covers the tip of the penis (glans). It is very important to keep the area beneath it clean.

Glands in the Male Reproductive System

Accessory Glands
The accessory glands of the male reproductive system are the seminal vesicles, prostate gland, and the bulbourethral glands. These glands secrete fluids that enter the urethra.

Seminal Vesicles
The paired seminal vesicles are saccular glands posterior to the urinary bladder. Each gland has a short duct that joins with the ductus deferens at the ampulla to form an ejaculatory duct, which then empties into the urethra. The fluid from the seminal vesicles is viscous and contains fructose, which provides an energy source for the sperm; prostaglandins, which contribute to the mobility and viability of the sperm; and proteins that cause slight coagulation reactions in the semen after ejaculation.

Prostate
The prostate gland is a firm, dense structure that is located just inferior to the urinary bladder. It is about the size of a walnut and encircles the urethra as it leaves the urinary bladder. Numerous short ducts from the substance of the prostate gland empty into the prostatic urethra. The secretions of the prostate are thin, milky colored, and alkaline. They function to enhance the motility of the sperm. (We will go in further detail about the prostate in the next chapter.)

Bulbourethral Glands

The paired bulbourethral (Cowper's) glands are small, about the size of a pea, and located near the base of the penis. A short duct from each gland enters the proximal end of the penile urethra. In response to sexual stimulation, the bulbourethral glands secrete an alkaline mucus-like fluid. This fluid neutralizes the acidity of the urine residue in the urethra, helps to neutralize the acidity of the vagina, and provides some lubrication for the tip of the penis during intercourse.

Seminal Fluid

Seminal fluid, or semen, is a slightly alkaline mixture of sperm cells and secretions from the accessory glands. Secretions from the seminal vesicles make up about 60 percent of the volume of the semen, with most of the remainder coming from the prostate gland. The sperm and secretions from the bulbourethral gland contribute only a small volume.

The volume of semen in a single ejaculation may vary from 1.5 to 6.0 ml. There are usually between 50 to 150 million sperm per milliliter of semen. Sperm counts below 10 to 20 million per milliliter usually present fertility problems. Although only one sperm actually penetrates and fertilizes the ovum, it takes several million sperm in an ejaculation to ensure that fertilization will take place.

Duct System
Sperm cells pass through a series of ducts to reach the outside of the body. After they leave the testes, the sperm passes through the epididymis, ductus deferens, ejaculatory duct, and urethra.

Epididymis
Sperm leave the testes through a series of efferent ducts that enter the epididymis. Each epididymis is a long (about 6 meters) tube that is tightly coiled to form a comma-shaped organ located along the superior and posterior margins of the testes. When the sperm leave the testes, they are immature and incapable of fertilizing ova. They complete their maturation process and become fertile as they move through the epididymis. Mature sperm are stored in the lower portion, or tail, of the epididymis.

Ductus Deferens
The ductus deferens, also called vas deferens, is a fibromuscular tube that is continuous (or contiguous) with the epididymis. It begins at the bottom (tail) of the epididymis then turns sharply upward along the posterior margin of the testes. The ductus deferens enters the abdominopelvic cavity through the inguinal canal and passes along the lateral pelvic wall. It crosses over the ureter and posterior portion of the urinary bladder, and then descends along the posterior wall of the bladder toward the prostate gland. Just before it reaches the prostate gland, each ductus deferens enlarges to form an ampulla. Sperm are stored in the proximal portion of the ductus deferens, near the epididymis, and

peristaltic movements propel the sperm through the tube.

The proximal portion of the ductus deferens is a component of the spermatic cord, which contains vascular and neural structures that supply the testes. The spermatic cord contains the ductus deferens, testicular artery and veins, lymph vessels, testicular nerve, cremaster muscle that elevates the testes for warmth and at times of sexual stimulation, and a connective tissue covering.

Ejaculatory Duct
Each ductus deferens, at the ampulla, joins the duct from the adjacent seminal vesicle (one of the accessory glands) to form a short ejaculatory duct. Each ejaculatory duct passes through the prostate gland and empties into the urethra.

Urethra
The urethra extends from the urinary bladder to the external urethral orifice at the tip of the penis. It is a passageway for sperm and fluids from the reproductive system and urine from the urinary system. While reproductive fluids are passing through the urethra, sphincters contract tightly to keep urine from entering the urethra.

The male urethra is divided into three regions. The prostatic urethra is the proximal portion that passes through the prostate gland. It receives the ejaculatory duct, which contains sperm and secretions from the seminal vesicles, and numerous ducts from the prostate glands. The next portion, the membranous urethra, is a short region that passes through the pelvic floor. The longest portion is the penile urethra (also called spongy urethra or cavernous urethra), which extends the length of the penis and opens to the outside at the external urethral orifice. The ducts from the bulbourethral glands open into the penile urethra.

Testes

The male gonads, testes or testicles, begin their development high in the abdominal cavity, near the kidneys. During the last two months before birth, or shortly after birth, they descend through the inguinal canal into the scrotum, a pouch that extends below the abdomen, posterior to the penis. Although this location of the testes, outside the abdominal cavity, may seem to make them vulnerable to injury, it provides a temperature about 3° C below normal body temperature. This lower temperature is necessary for the production of viable sperm.

Sagittal section of a testis and Epididymis

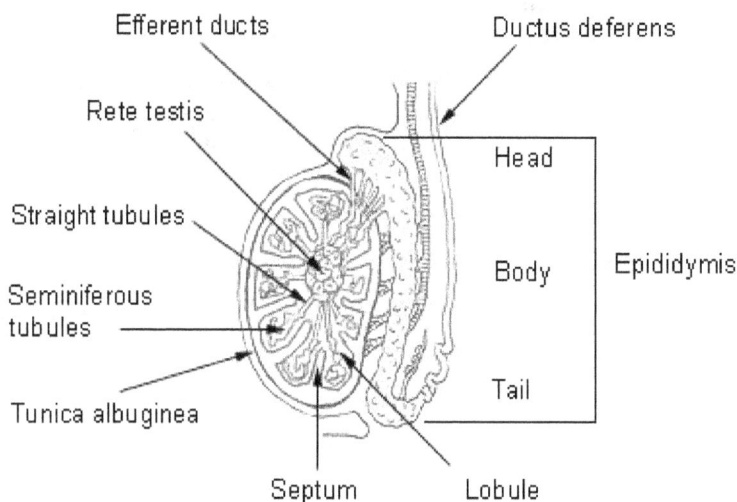

The scrotum consists of skin and subcutaneous tissue. A vertical septum, or partition, of subcutaneous tissue in the center divides it into two parts, each containing one testis. Smooth muscle fibers, called the dartos muscle, in the subcutaneous tissue contract to give the scrotum its wrinkled appearance. When these fibers are relaxed, the scrotum is smooth. Another muscle, the cremaster muscle, consists of skeletal muscle fibers and controls the position of the scrotum and testes. When it is cold or a man is sexually aroused, this muscle contracts to pull the testes closer to the body for warmth.

Scrotum/Testis/Balls

Each testis is an oval structure about 5 cm long and 3 cm in diameter. A tough, white fibrous connective tissue capsule, the tunica albuginea, surrounds each testis and extends inward to form septa that partition the organ into lobules. There are about 250 lobules in each testis. Each lobule contains 1 to 4 highly coiled seminiferous tubules that converge to form a single straight tubule, which leads into the rete testis. Short efferent ducts exit the testes. Interstitial cells (cells of Leydig), which produce male sex hormones, are located between the seminiferous tubules within a lobule.

Spermatogenesis

Sperm are produced by spermatogenesis within the seminiferous tubules. A transverse section of a seminiferous tubule shows that it is packed with cells in various stages of development. Interspersed with these cells, there are large cells that extend from the periphery of the tubule to the lumen. These large cells are the supporting, or sustentacular cells (Sertoli's cells), which support and nourish the other cells.

Early in embryonic development, primordial germ cells enter the testes and differentiate into spermatogonia, immature cells that remain dormant until puberty. Spermatogonia are diploid cells, each with 46 chromosomes (23 pairs) located around the periphery of the seminiferous tubules. At puberty, hormones stimulate these cells to begin dividing by mitosis. Some of the daughter cells produced by mitosis remain at the periphery as spermatogonia. Others are pushed toward the lumen, undergo some changes, and become primary spermatocytes. Because they are produced by mitosis, primary spermatocytes, like spermatogonia, are diploid and have 46 chromosomes.

Each primary spermatocytes goes through the first meiotic division, meiosis I, to produce two secondary spermatocytes, each with 23 chromosomes (haploid). Just prior to this division, the genetic material is replicated so that each chromosome consists of two strands, called chromatids, that are joined by a centromere. During meiosis I, one chromosome, consisting of two chromatids, goes to each secondary spermatocyte. In the second meiotic division, meiosis II, each secondary spermatocyte divides to produce two spermatids. There is no replication of genetic material in this division, but the centromere divides so that a single-stranded chromatid goes to each cell. As a result of the two meiotic divisions, each primary spermatocyte produces four spermatids. During spermatogenesis there are two cellular divisions, but only one replication of DNA so that each spermatid has 23 chromosomes (haploid), one from each pair in the original primary spermatocyte. Each successive stage in spermatogenesis is pushed toward the center of the tubule so that the more immature cells are at the periphery and the more differentiated cells are nearer the center.

Spermatogenesis (and oogenesis in the female) differs from mitosis because the resulting cells have only half the number of chromosomes as the original cell. When the sperm cell nucleus unites with an egg cell nucleus, the full number of chromosomes is restored. If sperm and egg cells were produced by mitosis, then each successive generation would have twice the number of chromosomes as the preceding one.

The final step in the development of sperm is called spermiogenesis. In this process, the spermatids formed from spermatogenesis become mature spermatozoa, or sperm. The mature sperm cell has a head, midpiece, and tail. The head, also called the nuclear region, contains the 23 chromosomes surrounded by a nuclear membrane. The tip of the head is covered by an acrosome, which contains enzymes that help the sperm penetrate the female gamete. The midpiece, metabolic region, contains mitochondria that provide adenosine triphosphate (ATP). The tail or locomotor region, uses a typical flagellum for locomotion. The sperm are released into the lumen of the seminiferous tubule and leave the testes. They then enter the epididymis where they undergo their final maturation and become capable of fertilizing a female gamete.

Sperm production begins at puberty and continues throughout the life of a male. The entire process, beginning with a primary spermatocyte, takes about 74 days. After ejaculation, the sperm can live for about 48 hours in the female reproductive tract.

Males, Diseases, and Ailments

What is Peyronie's disease?

Peyronie's disease is a disorder in which scar tissue, called a plaque, forms in the penis—the male organ used for urination and sex. The plaque builds up inside the tissues of a thick, elastic membrane called the tunica albuginea. The most common area for the plaque is on the top or bottom of the penis. As the plaque builds up, the penis will curve or bend, which can cause painful erections. Curves in the penis can make sexual intercourse painful, difficult, or impossible. Peyronie's disease begins with inflammation, or swelling, which can become a hard scar.

The plaque that develops in Peyronie's disease is not the same plaque that can develop in a person's arteries. The plaque seen in Peyronie's disease is benign, or noncancerous, and is not a tumor. Peyronie's disease is not contagious or caused by any known transmittable disease.

Early researchers thought Peyronie's disease was a form of impotence, now called erectile dysfunction (ED). ED happens when a man is unable to achieve or keep an erection firm enough for sexual intercourse. Some men with Peyronie's disease may have ED. Usually men with Peyronie's disease are referred to a urologist—a doctor who specializes in sexual and urinary problems.

How does an erection occur?

An erection occurs when blood flow increases into the penis, making it expand and become firm. Two long chambers inside the penis, called the corpora cavernosa, contain a spongy tissue that draws blood into the chambers. The spongy tissue contains smooth muscles, fibrous tissues, spaces, veins, and arteries. The tunica albuginea encases the corpora cavernosa. The urethra, which is the tube that carries urine and semen outside of the body, runs along the underside of the corpora cavernosa in the middle of a third chamber called the corpus spongiosum.

An erection requires a precise sequence of events:

- An erection begins with sensory or mental stimulation, or both. The stimulus may be physical contact or a sexual image or thought.

- When the brain senses a sexual urge, it sends impulses to local nerves in the penis that cause the muscles of the corpora cavernosa to relax. As a result, blood flows in through the arteries and fills the spaces in the corpora cavernosa like water filling a sponge.

- The blood creates pressure in the corpora cavernosa, making the penis expand.

- The tunica albuginea helps trap the blood in the corpora cavernosa, thereby sustaining the erection.

- The erection ends after climax or after the sexual urge has passed. The muscles in the penis contract to stop the inflow of blood. The veins open and the extra blood flows out of the penis and back into the body.

What causes Peyronie's disease?

Medical experts do not know the exact cause of Peyronie's disease. Many believe that Peyronie's disease may be the result of

- acute injury to the penis

- chronic, or repeated, injury to the penis

- autoimmune disease—a disorder in which the body's immune system attacks the body's own cells and organs

Injury to the Penis

Medical experts believe that hitting or bending the penis may injure the tissues inside. A man may injure the penis during sex, athletic activity, or an accident. Injury ruptures blood vessels, which leads to bleeding and swelling inside the layers of the tunica albuginea. Swelling inside the penis will block blood flow through the layers of tissue inside the penis. When the blood can't flow normally, clots can form and trap immune system cells. As the injury heals, the immune system cells may release substances that lead to the formation of too much scar tissue. The scar tissue builds up and forms a plaque inside the penis. The plaque reduces the elasticity of tissues and flexibility of the penis during erection, leading to curvature. The plaque may further harden because of calcification—the process in which calcium builds up in body tissue.

Autoimmune Disease

Some medical experts believe that Peyronie's disease may be part of an autoimmune disease. Normally, the immune system is the body's way of protecting itself from infection by identifying and destroying bacteria, viruses, and other potentially harmful foreign substances. Men who have autoimmune diseases may develop Peyronie's disease when the immune system attacks cells in the penis. This can lead to inflammation in the penis and can cause scarring. Medical experts do not know what causes autoimmune diseases. Some of the autoimmune diseases associated with Peyronie's disease affect connective tissues. Connective tissue is specialized tissue that supports, joins, or separates different types of tissues and organs of the body.

A Man's Cry for Health

Colon Cancer

Colon Cancer kills more people than any other malignancy except lung cancer. One in 20 Americans will develop colon cancer in his/her lifetime-usually after age 50. Tragically, 90% colorectal cancers can be avoided through early detection.

Colon cancer is rare in regions and *people where vegetables and grains make up the bulk of their diet,* however, it is most common in the United States and other western nations where the diet is largely based on meat.

A diet rich in fruits, vegetables, beans, and whole grains prevents colon cancer. The American Cancer Society recommends at least five servings of these foods per day. While it is hard to determine exactly which components of this healthy diet are protective, research has zeroed in on several candidates.

Breast Cancer in Men

The American Cancer Society estimates for breast cancer in men in the United States for 2017 are:
- About 2,470 new cases of invasive breast cancer in men will be diagnosed
- About 460 men will die from breast cancer

Breast cancer is about 100 times less common among men than among women. For men, the lifetime risk of getting breast cancer is about 1 in 1,000. The number of breast cancer cases in men relative to the population has been fairly stable over the last 30 years.

Bone Cancer

Primary bone cancer is cancer that starts in the bone. Less than 0.2% of all cancers are primary bone cancer. However, it is much more common for bones to be the site of metastasis or spread from other cancers. The statistics below are about primary bone cancer.

This year, an estimated 3,260 people of all ages (1,820 men and boys and 1,440 women and girls) in the United States will be diagnosed with primary bone cancer.

It is estimated that 1,550 deaths (890 men and boys and 660 women and girls) from this disease will occur this year.

In adults, chondrosarcoma makes up more than 35% of primary bone cancers, followed by osteosarcoma (22%), chordoma (10%), Ewing sarcoma (8%), and UPS/fibrosarcoma (4%). The remaining types of bone cancer are rare. In teens and children, osteosarcoma (56%) and Ewing sarcoma (34%) are much more common.

The 5-year survival rate tells you what percent of people live at least 5 years after the cancer is found. Percent means how many out of 100. The 5-year survival rate for people diagnosed with bone cancer at an early stage is about 85%. Around 40% of bone cancer is diagnosed at an early stage.
The 5-year survival rate for adult bone cancer is 66%. Adults with chondrosarcoma have a 5-year survival rate of 80% compared to a 5-year survival rate of 54% for osteosarcoma.

There are many ways to practice prevention with all disease, and these practices are a healthy diet rich in raw fruits and vegetables, as well as avoiding the foods that are saturated in sugar and other unhealthy fats. It is also extremely important to add exercise to our life. There are also herbs like chamomile, Black Walnut, and lavender that assist with pain and removing toxins from the colon.

The Health of the Prostate

The prostate gland makes fluid that forms part of semen. The prostate lies just below the bladder in front of the rectum. It surrounds the urethra (the tube that carries urine and semen through the penis and out of the body).

Prostate cancer is the most common cancer in men in the United States, after skin cancer. It is the second leading cause of death from cancer in men. Prostate cancer occurs more often in African-American men than in white men. African-American men with prostate cancer are more likely to die from the disease than white men with prostate cancer.

Almost all prostate cancers are adenocarcinomas (cancers that begin in cells that make and release mucus and other fluids). Prostate cancer often has no early symptoms. Advanced prostate cancer can cause men to urinate more often or have a weaker flow of urine, but these symptoms can also be caused by benign prostate conditions.

Prostate cancer usually grows very slowly. Most men with prostate cancer are older than 65 years and do not die from the disease. Finding and treating prostate cancer before symptoms occur may not improve health or help you live longer.

For men diagnosed with prostate cancer that has spread to other parts of the body, the 5-year survival rate is 30%. Prostate cancer is the second leading cause of cancer death in men in the United States. It is estimated that 29,430 deaths from this disease will occur this year.

Can Cigarettes & Alcohol Cause Erectile Dysfunction?

Erectile Dysfunction affects almost all men at some point of their lives. According to Sharecare, it affects as many as 30 million American men, including 30 to 50 percent of men between the ages of 40 and 70.

While many psychological and physical issues can contribute to ED, cigarette smoking can lead to permanent problems with erection because over time smoking can damage the blood vessels. For men under 40, it seems smoking cigarettes has become the major cause of ED. Cigarette smoke contains over 4,000 chemicals, including 43 known cancer causing (carcinogenic) compounds and 400 other toxins. These cigarette ingredients include nicotine, tar, carbon monoxide, formaldehyde, ammonia, cyanide, arsenic, and DDT.

Nicotine is very addictive, and the chemicals that coincide with the nicotine in your cigarettes are extremely harmful. Furthermore, if you can imagine for a moment that carbon monoxide, cyanide and formaldehyde are circulating in your blood stream each time you smoke a cigarette & then imagine it circulating to/in your penis. Over time, this chemical overload is not only damaging your body, but it is also killing the possibility of a proper erection. Unfortunately, the longer you continue to smoke cigarettes, the harder it becomes to reverse ED. There are other smoke options available besides choosing to consume 4000 chemicals per cigarette, but the absolute best option for a proper erection and your overall health is not to smoke at all.

Overindulging in alcoholic beverages can also contribute to ED. Even though alcohol seems to open up the courage and spontaneous box in most people, it is also known as a depressant and can cause liver toxicity. If the liver starts to suffer, all other organs including the penis will reap the harmful side effects.

One of the best things you can do to encourage a proper erection is eat healthier foods. Consuming more fruits and vegetables in their raw state can provide the body with all the nutrients while also encouraging better circulation to the organs. Exercise is another healthy contribution you can offer the penis, as it also contributes to better circulation to all the organs, including the penis. Since stress is also a restriction on the body, find proper ways to relieve tension in your body such as massages, yoga, and meditation. Nature also provides some of the best herbal remedies for ED.

What is Diabetes?

Diabetes is a disease that occurs when your blood glucose, also called blood sugar, is too high. Blood glucose is your main source of energy and comes from the food you eat. Insulin, a hormone made by the pancreas, helps glucose from food get into your cells to be used for energy. Sometimes your body doesn't make enough—or any—insulin or doesn't use insulin well. Glucose then stays in your blood and doesn't reach your cells.
Over time, having too much glucose in your blood can cause health problems.

Sometimes people call diabetes "a touch of sugar" or "borderline diabetes." These terms suggest that someone doesn't really have diabetes or has a less serious case, but every case of diabetes is serious.

What are the different types of diabetes?

The most common types of diabetes are type 1, type 2, and gestational diabetes.

Type 1 diabetes

If you have type 1 diabetes, your body does not make insulin. Your immune system attacks and destroys the cells in your pancreas that make insulin. Type 1 diabetes is usually diagnosed in children and young adults, although it can appear at any age.

Type 2 diabetes

If you have type 2 diabetes, your body does not make or use insulin well. You can develop type 2 diabetes at any age, even during childhood. However, this type of diabetes occurs most often in middle-aged and older people. Type 2 is the most common type of diabetes.

Gestational diabetes

Gestational diabetes develops in some women when they are pregnant. Most of the time, this type of diabetes goes away after the baby is born. However, if you've had gestational diabetes, you have a greater chance of developing type 2 diabetes later in life. Sometimes diabetes diagnosed during pregnancy is actually type 2 diabetes.

Other types of diabetes

Less common types include monogenic diabetes, which is an inherited form of diabetes, and cystic fibrosis-related diabetes.

How common is diabetes?

As of 2015, 30.3 million people in the United States, or 9.4 percent of the population, had diabetes. More than 1 in 4 of them didn't know they had the disease. Diabetes affects 1 in 4 people over the age of 65. About 90-95 percent of cases in adults are type 2 diabetes.

Who is more likely to develop type 2 diabetes?

You are more likely to develop type 2 diabetes if you are age 45 or older, have a family history of diabetes, or are overweight. Physical inactivity, race, and certain health problems such as high blood pressure also affect your chance of developing type 2 diabetes.

What health problems can people with diabetes develop?

Over time, high blood glucose leads to problems such as

- heart disease
- stroke
- kidney disease
- eye problems
- dental disease
- nerve damage
- foot problems

You can take steps to lower your chances of developing these diabetes-related health problems by approaching your health stresses holistically.

Diabetes & Sexual & Urologic Problems

Troublesome bladder symptoms and changes in sexual function are common health problems as people age. Having diabetes can mean early onset and increased severity of these problems. Sexual and urologic complications of diabetes occur because of the damage diabetes can cause to blood vessels and nerves. Men may have difficulty with erections or ejaculation. Women may have problems with sexual response and vaginal lubrication. Urinary tract infections and bladder problems occur more often in people with diabetes. People who keep their diabetes under control can lower their risk of the early onset of these sexual and urologic problems.

Diabetes and Sexual Problems

Both men and women with diabetes can develop sexual problems because of damage to nerves and small blood vessels. When a person wants to lift an arm or take a step, the brain sends nerve signals to the appropriate muscles. Nerve signals also control internal organs like the heart and bladder, but people do not have the same kind of conscious control over them as they do over their arms and legs. The nerves that control internal organs are called autonomic nerves, which signal the body to digest food and circulate blood without a person having to think about it. The body's response to sexual stimuli is also involuntary, governed by autonomic nerve signals that increase blood flow to the genitals and cause smooth muscle tissue to relax. Damage to these autonomic nerves can hinder normal function. Reduced blood flow resulting from damage to blood vessels can also contribute to sexual dysfunction.

Bladder Problems

Many events or conditions can damage nerves that control bladder function, including diabetes and other diseases, injuries, and infections. More than half of men and women with diabetes have bladder dysfunction because of damage to nerves that control bladder function. Bladder dysfunction can have a profound effect on a person's quality of life. Common bladder problems in men and women with diabetes include the following:

Overactive bladder. Damaged nerves may send signals to the bladder at the wrong time, causing its muscles to squeeze without warning. The symptoms of overactive bladder include

- urinary frequency-urination eight or more times a day or two or more times a night
- urinary urgency-the sudden, strong need to urinate immediately
- urge incontinence-leakage of urine that follows a sudden, strong urge to urinate

Poor control of sphincter muscles
Sphincter muscles surround the urethra-the tube that carries urine from the bladder to the outside of the body-and keep it closed to hold urine in the bladder. If the nerves to the sphincter muscles are damaged, the muscles may become loose and allow leakage or stay tight when a person is trying to release urine.

Urine Retention
For some people, nerve damage keeps their bladder muscles from getting the message that it is time to urinate or makes the muscles too weak to completely empty the bladder. If the bladder becomes too full, urine may back up and the increasing pressure may damage the kidneys.

If urine remains in the body too long, an infection can develop in the kidneys or bladder. Urine retention may also lead to overflow incontinence-leakage of urine when the bladder is full and does not empty properly.

Diagnosis of bladder problems may involve checking both bladder function and the appearance of the bladder's interior. Tests may include x-rays, urodynamic testing to evaluate bladder function, and cystoscopy, a test that uses a device called a cystoscope to view the inside of the bladder.

Treatment of bladder problems due to nerve damage depends on the specific problem. If the main problem is urine retention, treatment may involve medication to promote better bladder emptying and a practice called timed voiding-urinating on a schedule-to promote more efficient urination.

Sometimes people need to periodically insert a thin tube called a catheter through the urethra into the bladder to drain the urine. Learning how to tell when the bladder is full and how to massage the lower abdomen to fully empty the bladder can help as well.

If urinary leakage is the main problem, medications, strengthening muscles with Kegel exercises, or surgery can help. Treatment for the urinary urgency and frequency of overactive bladder may involve medications, timed voiding, Kegel exercises, and surgery in some cases.

Urinary Tract Infections
Infections can occur when bacteria, usually from the digestive system, reach the urinary tract. If bacteria are growing in the urethra, the infection is called urethritis. The bacteria may travel up the urinary tract and cause a bladder infection, called cystitis. An untreated infection may go farther into the body and cause pyelonephritis, a kidney infection. Some people have chronic or recurrent urinary tract infections. Symptoms of urinary tract infections can include

- a frequent urge to urinate
- pain or burning in the bladder or urethra during urination
- cloudy or reddish urine
- in women, pressure above the pubic bone
- in men, a feeling of fullness in the rectum

If the infection is in the kidneys, a person may have nausea, feel pain in the back or side, and have a fever. Frequent urination can be a sign of high blood glucose, so results from recent blood glucose monitoring should be evaluated.

The health care provider will ask for a urine sample, which will be analyzed for bacteria and pus.

Additional tests may be done if the patient has frequent urinary tract infections. An ultrasound exam provides images from the echo patterns of sound waves bounced back from internal organs. An intravenous pyelogram uses a special dye to enhance x-ray images of the urinary tract. Cystoscopy might be performed.

Early diagnosis and treatment are important to prevent more serious infections. To clear up a urinary tract infection, the health care provider will probably prescribe antibiotic treatment based on the type of bacteria in the urine. Kidney infections are more serious and may require several weeks of antibiotic treatment. Drinking plenty of fluids will help prevent another infection.

Heart Disease

Heart Disease Facts in Men
- Heart disease is the leading cause of death for men in the United States, killing 321,000 men in 2013—that's **1 in every 4** male deaths.[1]
- Heart disease is the **leading cause** of death for men of most racial/ethnic groups in the United States, including African Americans, American Indians or Alaska Natives, Hispanics, and whites. For Asian American or Pacific Islander men, heart disease is second only to cancer.[2]
- About 8.5% of all white men, 7.9% of black men, and 6.3% of Mexican American men have coronary heart disease.[3]

- **Half** of the men who die suddenly of coronary heart disease have **no previous symptoms**.[3] Even if you have no symptoms, you may still be at risk for heart disease.
- **Between 70% and 89%** of sudden cardiac events occur in men.[3]

Risk Factors
High blood pressure, high LDL (bad) cholesterol, and smoking are key risk factors for heart disease. About **half of Americans** (49%) have at least one of these three risk factors.

Several other medical conditions and lifestyle choices can also put people at a higher risk for heart disease, including:
- Diabetes
- Overweight and obesity
- Poor diet
- Physical inactivity
- Excessive alcohol use

Heart attack

A heart attack (myocardial infarction) occurs when a plaque ruptures, allowing a blood clot to form, which can be life-threatening. The blood clot completely obstructs the artery, stopping blood flow to part of the heart muscle, and that portion of muscle dies.
Abnormal heart rhythms and sudden cardiac arrest
The heart is an electrical pump composed of heart muscle and cells that produce and conduct electrical signals. Heart muscle cells can become irritable

because they have lost blood supply and may, in addition, cause electrical abnormalities or short circuits that prevent the heart muscle from pumping which can result in sudden cardiac death.

Heart disease risk factors

The major risk factors for heart disease (and stroke and peripheral vascular disease) include smoking, high blood pressure, high cholesterol, diabetes, and family history.

Angina
The coronary arteries are at risk for narrowing as cholesterol deposits, called plaques, build up inside the artery. If the arteries narrow enough, blood supply to the heart muscle may be compromised (slowed down), and this slowing of blood flow to the heart causes pain, or angina.
Angina symptoms include:
chest pressure with radiation down the arm and to the jaw, shortness of breath, sweating, indigestion, nausea, a decreased ability to do routine activities.
This heart pain is often referred to as "anginal equivalent."

The Best foods for Heart Health (see 104-121)

Stroke (cerebrovascular accident, CVA)

A stroke (cerebrovascular accident [CVA]), occurs when blood supply to part of the brain is disrupted, causing brain cells to die. Blood flow can be compromised by a variety of mechanisms. This can occur because blood supply has been cut off (ischemia) or because there has been bleeding in the brain (hemorrhage). Ischemic strokes occur due to a variety of reasons including the gradual narrowing of a blood vessel in the brain, debris that can break off from the carotid artery in the neck, or from a blood clot that embolizes (or travels) from the heart.

The risk factors for stroke are the same as for heart disease: smoking, high blood pressure, high cholesterol, and family history.

A TIA (transient ischemic attack, mini-stroke) is a stroke that improves, usually quickly. A person develops stroke like symptoms (weakness of one side of the body or face, vision loss, speech difficulty) but it resolves spontaneously within a few minutes or hours. This situation should never be ignored since it is a major warning sign that an impending stroke may occur.

COPD

Emphysema and chronic bronchitis are the two types of chronic obstructive pulmonary disease (COPD) and both are most commonly caused by smoking. Due to the toxins in smoke, the lung tissue is damaged and loses its ability to transfer oxygen from the inhaled air into the blood stream. Symptoms of

COPD include shortness of breath and wheezing. COPD increases the risk of lung infection including pneumonia.

Influenza and pneumonia
A healthy lifestyle and healthy body makes for a strong immune system that can fight common infections like influenza (flu). It is important to follow public health recommendations for routine immunizations to reduce the risk of contracting the flu, and its complications such as pneumonia. However, pneumonia is not limited to just viral causes. Bacterial pneumonia is ranked with influenza as one of the major causes of death in men by many researchers.

Suicide
Thoughts of self harm are not normal. They should not be ignored by a man, family, or friends, and should be considered an emergency situation. Depression can become overwhelming and potentially life-threatening. Men with depression may be able to function reasonably well on a day to day basis and may be reluctant to seek help. It may take a crisis situation to finally get a man to agree to get medical, psychological, and counseling assistance.

Symptoms of depression may be subtle and arise slowly. They can include:
- difficulty concentrating or completing projects
- lack of energy

- difficulty sleeping or sleeping too much
- change in appetite (some people stop eating while others overeat)
- feelings of hopelessness or worthlessness
- excessive sadness or feelings of emptiness
- thoughts of suicide or self harm

Kidney disease
The kidneys filter impurities from the blood and dispose of them in the urine. They are also important in maintaining electrolyte balance in the blood. Even in healthy people, aging gradually decreases the efficiency of kidney function. Kidney failure is often a result of years of poorly controlled high blood pressure and diabetes.
In the United States, approximately 26 million people have chronic kidney disease.

Alzheimer's disease
Dementia and Alzheimer's disease describes a gradual loss of cognition and intellectual ability including language, attention, memory, and problem solving is an otherwise healthy person. The cause is unknown and there is no cure. Recommendations to decrease the risk of dementia include avoiding smoking, and keeping blood pressure, high cholesterol, and diabetes under control. Physical and mental fitness may help prevent dementia; keeping socially active may also help. Recurrent head injuries are associated with dementia. Alzheimer's disease and dementia are not direct causes of death, but they make it more difficult to identify and treat complications that can lead to death.

Sugar

We have all at some point of our lives have been introduced to the sweetest legal drug known to man, which is mainly refined white sugar. We have celebrated Halloween and collected candy from all our friendly neighbors, and no one ever told us, "Sugar is a drug so you shouldn't eat it," or," Sugar can cause many diseases in your body, so don't eat it."

According to Dr. David Reuben, author of "Everything You Always Wanted to Know About Nutrition says,

White refined sugar-is not a food. It is a pure chemical extracted from plant sources, purer in fact than cocaine, which it resembles in many ways.

Its true name is sucrose and its chemical formula is $C12H22O11$. It has 12 carbon atoms, 22 hydrogen atoms, 11 oxygen atoms, and absolutely nothing else to offer." ...The chemical formula for cocaine is $C17H21NO4$. Sugar's formula again is $C12H22O11$. For all practical purposes, the difference is that sugar is missing the "N", or nitrogen atom. ...Refining means to make "pure" by a process of extraction or separation. Sugars are refined by taking a natural food, which contains a high percentage of sugar, and then removing all elements of that food until only the sugar remains. ...While sugar is commonly made from sugar cane or sugar beets. Through heating and mechanical and chemical processing, all vitamins, minerals, proteins, fats, enzymes and indeed every nutrient is removed until only the sugar remains. Sugar cane and sugar beets are first harvested and then chopped into small pieces, squeezing out the juice, which is then mixed with water. This liquid is then heated, and lime is added.

After the crystals condense, they are bleached snow-white usually by the use of pork or cattle bones. ...During the refining process, 64 food elements are destroyed. All the potassium, magnesium, calcium, iron, manganese, phosphate, and sulfate are removed. The A, D, and B, vitamins are destroyed.

I read of a study done on rats and sugar. In the study, the scientist first made sure that the rats were addicted to cocaine. After the assured the cocaine addiction, they started the rats on refined sugar until the rats were addicted to sugar.
 Once the scientist were able to confirm both addictions, they placed the cocaine in one corner of a cage, and they placed sugar in the other corner of the cage. When the rats were released, every single rat ran to the sugar.

Are you addicted to sugar?

Cancer and Sugar Connection
Patrick Quillin, PHD, RD, CNS, former director of nutrition for Cancer Treatment Centers of America in Tulsa, OK, wrote: "It puzzles me why the simple concept 'sugar feeds cancer' can be so dramatically overlooked as part of a comprehensive cancer treatment plan" (*Nutrition Science News,* April 2000) Here are reasons that cancer and sugar are best friends.

1-Affinity
Cancer cells love sugar! That is why refined carbohydrates like white sugar, white flour, high fructose corn syrup (HFCS) and soft drinks are extremely dangerous for anyone trying to prevent or reverse cancer. Sugar essentially feeds tumors and encourages cancer growth. Cancer cells uptake sugar at 10-12 times the rate of healthy cells. In fact, that is the basis of PET (positron emission tomography) scans -- one of the most accurate tools for detecting cancer growth. PET scans use radioactively labeled glucose to detect sugar-hungry tumor cells. When patients drink the sugar water, it gets preferentially taken up into the cancer cells and they light up! The 1931 Nobel laureate in medicine, German Otto Warburg, PhD, discovered that cancer cells have a fundamentally different energy metabolism compared to healthy cells. He found that malignant tumors exhibit increased glycolysis -- a process whereby glucose is used as a fuel by cancer -- as compared with normal cells.

2-Acidity
Warburg also found that cancers thrive in an acidic environment. Sugar is highly acidic. With a pH of about 6.4, it is 10 times more acidic than the ideal alkaline pH of blood at 7.4.

3-Immunity
Sugar suppresses a key immune response known as phagocytosis – the Pac-Man effect of the immune system. Consuming 10 teaspoons of sugar can cause about a 50% reduction in phagocytosis. If you consider the sugar in your cereal, the syrup on your waffles and pancakes, the sugar added to your morning coffee or tea, the sugar in cold beverages like iced tea or lemonade, the HFCS in prepared foods, salad dressing and ketchup, and of course sugary snacks and desserts, you can see how easy it is to suppress your immune systems significantly. Not only the amount of sugar, but also the frequency of ingesting sugar is relevant to immune function. In one study, research subjects were found to have nearly a 38% decrease in phagocytosis one hour after ingesting a moderate amount of sugar. Two hours later, the immune system was suppressed 44%; immune function did not recover completely for a full five hours.

4-Activity
In most people, when sugar in any form is consumed, the pancreas releases insulin. Breast tissue, for example, contains insulin receptors, and insulin is a powerful stimulant of cell growth. One group of Australian researchers concluded that high levels of

insulin and insulin-like growth factor (IGF) may actually be causative of cancers of the breast, prostate, endometrium and pancreas. A broad study conducted in 21 countries in Europe, North America and Asia concluded that sugar intake is a strong risk factor contributing to higher breast cancer rates, particularly in older women. A four-year study at the National Institute of Public Health and Environmental Protection in the Netherlands compared 111 biliary tract cancer patients with 480 healthy controls. Sugar intake was associated with more than double the cancer risk.

5- Obesity
Sugar ingestion seriously contributes to obesity, a known cause of cancer. Obesity also negatively affects survival. More than 100,000 cases of cancer each year are caused by excess body fat, according to the American Institute for Cancer research. These include esophageal, pancreatic, kidney, gallbladder, breast and colorectal cancer.

Different types of sweeteners.

Corn Syrup: Made from corn and usually 100% glucose. According to the Food and Drug Administration (FDA), "corn syrup" can be used to describe numerous corn-derived products.

Fructose: A simple sugar found in fruits, honey, and root vegetables. It is used as a caloric sweetener, added to foods and beverages in the form of crystalline fructose (made from corn starch), and it makes up about half the sugar in sucrose or high fructose corn syrup (see below). Fructose does not elicit a glycemic response so it sometimes has been used as a sweetener for foods intended for people with diabetes. However, because of concern about the effect of excessive use on blood lipids, the Academy of Nutrition and Dietetics does not recommend fructose as a sweetening agent for people with diabetes.

Galactose: A simple sugar found in milk and dairy foods. Galactose and glucose form the disaccharide lactose.

Glucose: The main source of energy for the body and the only used by brain cells. Glucose is produced when carbohydrates are digested or metabolized. Glucose is sometimes referred to as dextrose. Starch is comprised of long chains of glucose. Glucose make up exactly half of the sugar in sucrose and nearly half of the sugar in high fructose corn syrup.

A Man's Cry for Health

Philosophy given to me on Sugar Addiction
We have become addicted to sugar as a nation and it is a direct result of our feeling of a lack of love for others, and ourselves as well as our lack of control over our emotions. We live in a world that has always rewarded us with sugary treats, and every holiday is celebrated with cakes, pies, and love. Also, our parents have often given us sweet treats to stop us from crying. Now, when we are saddened or disturbed, we crave the thing that was a substitution for attention and love.

My Thoughts on Sugar and Substitutes
Instead of constantly trying to find substitutions for our sweet tooth addiction, we need to get over the addiction of thinking that everything needs to be sweet! Most fruits are naturally sweet, and before we eat foods to satisfy our cravings, we should eat the fruits of the earth. Now, if you have been advised to not eat certain fruits because of your blood sugar levels, there are plenty more fruits that you can enjoy.

I do not believe in sugar substitutions that degrade the body. Aspartame has been related to headaches, ADHD, Multiple Sclerosis, Seizures, Cancer and more. It is in some artificial sweeteners in the grocery stores.

According to the New Hampshire Department of Health & Human Services, the average American consumes almost 152 pounds of sugar in one year. This is equal to 3 pounds (or 6 cups) of sugar consumed in one week! Can you imagine eating 6 cups of straight sugar per week? When I imagined consuming only white, processed sugar, the thought makes me feel disgusted.

Bottom Line: The maximum amount of sugar consumption that is suggested per day by the American Heart Association for men is 9 teaspoons. Women, 6 teaspoons.

How many teaspoons of sugar are in one can of Coke? 10

We must work on discipline in regards to the things we decide to put in our mouth. Each teaspoon is either building or destroying our life, literally.

Sugar, Diet, and Mental Health
According to a study done on overall sugar consumption in 2002, a Dr. Arthur Westover, from the University of Texas Southwestern Medical Center in Dallas suspected sugar as a factor in higher rates of major depression.

Other research teams have looked into this concept and also discovered that eating not only sugar products, but also consuming fast food such as pizza, hamburgers, and other processed foods was found to increase depression.

Men with high sugar intakes have an increased likelihood of common mental disorders (such as anxiety and depression) after 5 years compared to those with low intakes, according to UCL research. The study also showed that having a mood disorder did not make people more inclined to eat foods with a high sugar content.

Anika Knüppel (UCL Institute of Epidemiology and Public Health), lead author of the paper said: "High sugar diets have a number of influences on our health but our study shows that there might also be a link between sugar and mood disorders, particularly among men. There are numerous factors that influence chances for mood disorders, but having a diet high in sugary foods and drinks might be the straw that breaks the camel's back.

Brittian has passed a tax law in April of 2018 that raised the taxes on soft drinks. Professor Eric

Brunner (UCL Institute of Epidemiology and Public Health) said, The physical and mental health of British people deserves some protection from the commercial forces which exploit the human 'sweet tooth.'

Spirit Talk: When we eat the foods of the earth, we ground ourselves with nature's first form of energy and we saturate our blood with the same nutrients that grow the earth. When we eat foods in their natural state, we give the earth our respect.

Processed sugar is literally a drug that our body loves, and though it contributes to every form of disease known to man, it is legal. Our teeth will also let us know when we have too much sugar in our system, because they start to 'ache' and decay.

We have to love ourselves enough to do right by our body. This is why it is so important to listen to our inner guides and be obedient to its advice. The more we ignore our inner voice, the more we teach ourselves that it is okay to disrespect ourselves.

Depression in Men

Almost every adult has felt pain and suffering at some point in their life. Whether it be the loss of a loved one, sexual abuse, racism, physical or mental abuse, etc., we have learned to internally mask our pain and deal with the repercussions on a superficial level. The reality is, when we internalize our saddened and negative emotions we end up expressing the pain in another form. These other options of expression may include one actually becoming an abuser because the process of releasing pain is difficult for some individuals. Until the person addresses their issues of dealing with abuse, they can become abusers of narcotics, alcohol, and people as a form of release.

For men in particular, releasing emotions are extremely difficult, because as a child he is taught that tears are a sign of weakness. However, when speaking on this subject with one of my male spiritual teachers, he said,

"If men were not meant to cry, we wouldn't have tear ducts."

~Jabade Powell

Tears serve as a release to our souls. We are constantly bombarded with family, life, and health stresses, on top of the challenging thoughts that we internally inflict on ourselves. Tears are another way to let go of all the negative burdens our spirit has to carry.

According to BeyondBlue.org, men suffer from depression for some of the following reasons:

Life events
Research suggests that continuing difficulties – long-term unemployment, living in an abusive or uncaring relationship, long-term isolation or loneliness, prolonged work stress – are more likely to cause depression than recent life stresses. However, recent events (such as losing your job) or a combination of events can 'trigger' depression if you're already at risk because of previous bad experiences or personal factors.

Family history
Depression can run in families and some people will be at an increased genetic risk. However, having a parent or close relative with depression doesn't mean you'll automatically have the same experience. Life circumstances and other personal factors are still likely to have an important influence.

Personality
Some people may be more at risk of depression because of their personality, particularly if they have a tendency to worry a lot, have low self-esteem, are perfectionists, are sensitive to personal criticism, or are self-critical and negative.

Serious medical illness

The stress and worry of coping with a serious illness can lead to depression, especially if you are dealing with long-term management and/or chronic pain.

Drug and alcohol use
Drug and alcohol use can both lead to and result from depression. Many people with depression also have drug and alcohol problems.

Spirit Talk: We often live in our thoughts verses living in the present moment, and it is our thoughts that predict our mood. We all have imagined the worst possibilities in our life, but we must acknowledge that our thoughts are only imagination and not truths. In this current reality, the world is bombarded with negativity, because many of us live in unpeaceful thoughts, thus creating an unhealthy vibration that radiates within most of humanity. At some point of our life, we have all experienced sadness and sorrow. When we continue to think about/imagine the situations that cause sorrow, we experience depression. Changing the way we think sounds like an easy task, but it is a process of undoing years of trained thinking habits that have become a part of who we are. Joe Dispenza wrote a book called, "Breaking the Habit of Being Yourself," and I suggest that everyone read this book, because it tackles the concept of undoing our thought patterns. We do not have to suffer in depression, and pharmaceutical medication is not the long-term answer. We are our own answer.

Addiction Statistics in America
- Over 20 million Americans over the age of 12 have an addiction (excluding tobacco).
- 100 people die every day from drug overdoses. This rate has tripled in the past 20 years.
- Over 5 million emergency room visits in 2011 were drug related.
- 2.6 million people with addictions have a dependence on both alcohol and illicit drugs.
- 9.4 million people in 2011 reported driving under the influence of illicit drugs.
- 6.8 million people with an addiction have a mental illness.
- Rates of illicit drug use is highest among those aged 18 to 25.
- Over 90% of those with an addiction began drinking, smoking or using illicit drugs before the age of 18.

Alcohol Statistics
- Binge drinking is more common in men; 9.1% of men 12 and older reported heavy drinking 5 or more days in a month, while 2.6% of women reported this.
- Over 11% of Americans have driven under the influence.
- Out of 16.6 million people with alcoholism, 2.6 million were also dependent on an illicit substance.

- It is estimated that over 95% of those who need treatment for alcoholism do not feel they need treatment.
- More people receive treatment for alcohol than any other substance.
- Over 30% of those who received treatment in 2011 reported using public or private health insurance to pay for treatment.

Tobacco and Nicotine Statistics

- Tobacco-related costs for the United States is over $190 billion (healthcare costs, loss of productivity, etc.)
- The rate of illicit drug use was 9.5 times higher in 2011 for teens who smoked cigarettes than those who didn't.
- Tobacco causes more deaths each year than all other substance abuse related deaths combined.
- Tobacco users in general are more likely to abuse drugs and alcohol. Over 40% of cigarette smokers reported binge drinking in 2011.
- The rates of pack-a-day smokers among those aged 18 to 25 has decreased by over 13% since 2002. ~Addiction Center

A Man's Cry for Health

Prescription Drugs and the Music Industry

Lately in the music industry, young rappers have glorified the idea of using pharmaceutical drugs to get high. Artist like Lil Zan (Zanax), Future, and many more constantly talk about intoxication with pharmaceutical drugs. A young rapper name Lil Peep made major headline news by overdosing on fentanyl, Xanax, marijuana, cocaine, Tramadol, hydrocodone, generic Dilaudid, oxycodone and oxymorphone, the majority of them being prescription drugs.

Another drug that has been glorified is codeine. Most hip-hop artists call it Syrup. A group named 36 Mafia from Memphis, Tennessee created a song called, "Sippin on some Sizzurp," which promoted the idea of drinking cough syrup to get high. Even though 36 Mafia was the first group to make a song about drinking cough syrup to get high, Houston Texas is where I first learned about drinking "Lean" aka Syrup.

Lean—also known as *purple drank*, *purple lean*, *sizzurp*, *dirty sprite*, and *lean drink*—is a combination of the following:
- Prescription-strength cough medicine (codeine).
- Soft drinks.
- Hard, fruit-flavored candy.

The prescription cough syrups used to make lean drink present the most danger because they often contain **codeine**, a powerful opioid drug. Another active ingredient in some prescription cough syrups is **promethazine,** an antihistamine that causes sedative effects and can impair motor functioning.

Suicidal Thoughts
According to the American Foundation of Suicide Prevention, 44,965 Americans die each year by suicide making suicide the 10th leading cause of death in the United States. Even though the average death by suicide in the United States is 123 people per day, Men die by suicide **3.53x** more often than women do.

I would be lying if I told you that I never thought about suicide, especially as a teen. The problems of my world just seemed unbearable, and the thought of permanently taking myself out of my vicious cycle of depression was an attractive thought. At one point in my teenage years, I even attempted to kill myself because I failed to realize that whatever I was going through was temporary.

When I was speaking with my sun/son about the concept of suicide, he said,

> "To actually try and kill yourself takes a lot of guts, because there is something in us that doesn't want to die."

Spirit Talk:

Life is not about a guaranteed emotion. As humans, we are subjected to joy, pain, sorrow, shame, etc. However, the emotions we go through in life allow us to dive deeper into self-awareness. Many of us look at the results of pain and sorrow in our life as if it is a curse, because it is hard to see the lesson our pain will carry while we are in the midst of the thing that is causing pain. The truth is, all emotions are temporary. If you are experiencing sadness, it is only a moment in time and you must understand that it will pass.

Our emotions are literally like the patterns of weather we experience on earth. On a bright sunny day, it can reflect an emotion of happiness and joy, feeling like an enchanted presence lives within us. More so, sadness and chaos can be a symbolism of storms, bringing rain in our life to help us grow and elevate into a better version of ourselves if we will allow. We are a reflection of nature, growing from our emotions as if seeds planted in the ground. The biggest lesson we need to remember is that we are allowed to feel the pain without being engulfed in the emotion.

Depression is real, and even though I am not a licensed psychologist, I believe depression comes from not being able to shake ourselves out of a destructive thinking pattern. In grade school, we were never taught about the importance of not allowing our negative thoughts to control our reality. So, when we are stuck in these thoughts of hopelessness and despair, it can become overbearing because we have not learned how to shed the feeling.

I want to tell you that life gets better. You have the power within you to change your circumstances no matter what you are facing. Even if it looks like there is no way out, you must embrace change and understand that you are God-Bodied, and as you go "through" your challenges, you will come out stronger because of them.

Your inner spirit/God/Source talks to you all the time. It tells you to be patient when you are rushing, to calm yourself when you are upset, and even to cheer up when you are sad. Our biggest issue is we have developed habitual thinking patterns of worry, fear and other negative vibrations that contribute to suffocating the peace we should always carry in our soul.

You are loved my friend. I hope most of all, when the dark clouds approach your life again, that you will embrace the rain and look at the wonderful opportunity to grow. I hope you will allow your higher self to direct your choices when your lower self seeks to fill a void by getting you addicted to drugs, food, or anything that leads to self-destruction.

Cherish your life my love. We need you.

Men and Chemicals

I wrote on this subject in my first book, Chemical Suicide/ Death by Association. The same chemicals in beauty and grooming products that are harmful to women are also harmful to men, but there is one chemical in particular that is harmful to men, and it is in almost everything.

Phthalates

Phthalates are in lots of products to make them flexible. PVC, cosmetics, cologne, hospitals, and almost anything that is plastic based. Even though phthalates are used in many different ways, they are horrible for your health. In men, high phthalate levels can cause sluggish sperm and low androgen levels. So if you are truly interests in going half on a baby with your mate, avoid the cologne, scented candles, stop heating your food in plastic, and please remove the pine scented air freshener from your rear view mirror.

Phthalates are banned in Europe because of the harsh side effects. In rodent studies, overexposure to phthalates have caused reproductive birth defects, and can cause genital deformities in your unborn seed.

Condoms and Chemicals

It is disturbing to even think about the idea that condoms can be hazardous to both you and your mate's health, but according to the national institute of health, the chemicals called N-Nitrosamines are potent carcinogens, and carry the potential to cause cervical cancer in your mate. Nitrosamines are a type of chemical found in tobacco products and tobacco smoke. Nitrosamines are also found in many foods, including fish, beer, fried foods, and meats. Some nitrosamines cause cancer in laboratory animals and may increase the risk of certain types of cancer in humans. Previously, endogenous nitrosamine formation in the vagina has been suggested as a cause of cervical cancer. It was speculated that exogenous N-nitrosamines and N-nitrosatable compounds from condoms may also lead to genital cancer. Research also suggested that the chances are low, but if your lubricants of choice are also carrying carcinogens, and you are heating up this unnatural concoction, it may be wiser to purchase condoms that are a healthier, vegan choice, such as Sir Richards condoms, Glyde condoms, Sustain, and a few more if you search the internet.

How Emotions Change the Organs

Heart: The heart, being the principal organ of the Vital Faculty, is very sensitive to emotional states. Noble, expansive, uplifting emotions like courage, valor, honesty, forthrightness, altruism and compassion strengthen the heart and Vital Spirits, whereas ignoble, constrictive, base emotions like cowardice, timidity, guilt, remorse, deceit and duplicity weaken them. Love and the emotional will to live are also very important to the heart; according to Greek Medicine, you CAN die of a broken heart. The heart, being the hottest organ in the body, is also very vulnerable to hot, turbulent passions, which can agitate the Vital Spirits to such an extent that they create a fever, which can be quite high and acute; Greek Medicine calls these fevers of energetic or emotional origin ephemeral fevers.

Lungs: The lungs, being an important noble organ of the Vital Faculty that works closely together with the heart, are sensitive and vulnerable to many of the same emotional states as the heart, and respond similarly. The lungs need a feeling of psychic space within which to function; the phrase, "breathing room" is a common expression. The feeling of being smothered, invalidated, or denied one's psychic space can constrict the lungs and cause respiratory problems like dyspnea and asthma. Conversely, a feeling of dignity and pride puffs up the chest, and allows the lungs to expand and function properly. Negative emotions that sap the will to live are also injurious to the lungs, especially grief and bereavement; many chronic respiratory diseases and conditions develop after a major loss or bereavement.

Throat: The throat is the body's main communications center, and is connected with the Throat Canter, or chakra. An inability to come out and speak one's truth will often cause physical problems with the throat; in extreme cases, one may even become mute and unable to speak. The throat is also the upper end of the digestive tract, and hence part of the Natural Faculty. Acute emotional tensions and anxieties can agitate the Natural Force in the liver, causing it to rise and get bottlenecked in the throat; one then feels like one's choking on something, or has something lodged in the throat, a condition called **globus hystericus**. Emotional gushings or catharses of sadness, grief or intense sentimentality will also cause a lump in the throat. Stuffing one's emotions and feelings down one's throat is injurious to its health, and will increase its vulnerability to dysfunction and disease.

Liver, Gall Bladder: Bile is produced by the liver and stored in the gall bladder, which makes these two organs vulnerable to negative Choleric emotions like anger, irritability, frustration, resentment, jealousy and envy. These negative Choleric emotions are stored in these organs, and can slowly eat away at them if allowed to fester. Anger and rage can explode upwards from the liver into the head, causing a lot of havoc in their wake: headaches, migraines; red, sore,

97

bloodshot eyes; and muscular tension in the neck and shoulders. Nervous and emotional tension and stress, as well as Melancholic emotions like pensiveness and worry, will stagnate the flow of the Natural Force in the liver, which in turn causes nervous, colicky, Melancholic disturbances of the digestive functions. This excess melancholy often accumulates under the lower ribs, whole giving a stuffy, distended, congested feeling in the chest and diaphragm area. This is the origin of the term *hypochondriac.*

Stomach: The stomach is a seething cauldron of emotions, and is intimately connected to the Gastric Center, or chakra, also called the Abdominal Center, which governs energy flow and distribution throughout the belly and gut. Choleric emotions like anger, hate, rage and frustration stored here lead to gastritis, ulcers and other Choleric stomach conditions. Many of us hold a lot of Choleric emotions like anger and resentment in our gut. Melancholic emotional stress and tension, as well as pensiveness, worry and anxiety, will stagnate the flow of the Natural Force in the stomach, causing distension, bloating, colic, gas and stomachache. And so, we must always try to be of good cheer when we eat. If accumulated Choleric and Melancholic emotional tensions in the stomach and Gastric Center get very severe, we may experience anorexia, appetite disorders, giddiness, nausea and dry heaves.

Spleen: The spleen is the storage receptacle for black bile. Therefore, it is adversely affected by negative Melancholic emotions like pensiveness, anxiety, worry and depression, which unduly constrict the free flow of the Natural Force through the digestive system and aggravate the Retentive Virtue, producing colic, gas, distension and bloating throughout the entire abdominal area. Actually a trio of subdiaphragmatic digestive organs can be adversely affected by negative Melancholic emotional states: the liver on the right, the spleen on the left, and the stomach in the middle.

Intestines and Bowels: The intestines are often the effect of psychosomatic or emotionally induced digestive disorders that arise in the upper digestive organs - the liver, gall bladder, stomach and spleen. The upper small intestine, or **duodenum**, being very close to these upper digestive organs, is the part most affected; these emotional disturbances are usually of a Choleric or Melancholic nature. In the middle and lower intestinal tract, Melancholic emotional disturbances are most injurious and keenly felt, because they aggravate the Retentive Virtue, producing colic and kinks in the intestines, or obstructions to their smooth flow and function.

Colon: Since the balanced, proper action of black bile is important to proper colon function, the colon is very vulnerable to aggravations and excesses of the Melancholic emotions - especially chronic or deeply held worry, anxiety and nervous or emotional stress and tension. Security issues and deep insecurities will also impact negatively on the colon, since its functioning is intimately connected with the Root Center, or chakra, which pertains to our emotional security. These Melancholic emotional disturbances usually produce disorders like constipation, irritable bowel syndrome, or spastic colon, but if the aggravation is severe, even colitis and more serious degenerative diseases may result.

Kidneys: Fright, fear and shock are most injurious to the kidneys. The energetic flow of these emotions is downwards, as they take away the foundation of security and self-assurance that we have. This also concerns the Root Center, or chakra, that root support or energetic foundation of strength and security that we have, which is closely connected to the kidneys and their balanced retention and evacuation of urine. When beset with extreme fear or fright, many lose control of their kidneys and bladder, and urinate spontaneously.

Adrenal glands: The adrenal glands, sitting right on top of the kidneys, are injured and drained energetically by excessive stress. The adrenal medulla and its fight-or-flight adrenaline response is excessively provoked by acute stress and emotional outbursts of anger and the like in those whose lives have become an overdramatized emotional roller coaster. Chronic stress aggravates the functioning of the adrenocortical hormones like cortisol, which can lead to weight gain, especially in the lower body and midriff, as well as rising blood sugar, if the stress is constant and unresolved. Since the adrenal glands provide the energetic support for healthy urinary function, the health, vitality and functioning of the kidneys will also be drained, and adversely affected by weakened or challenged adrenals.

Male Reproductive Organs: Since the male reproductive organs are closely linked, both functionally and anatomically, to the kidneys and urinary tract, negative emotions that adversely affect the kidneys, like fear, fright, shock and anxiety, will adversely affect male sexual function as well. Male impotence or sexual dysfunction, doesn't always have a physical cause; it can also be emotionally or psychosomatically induced by feelings of fear, inadequacy, insecurity or performance anxiety, which often operate on a subliminal level. Since the main energetic flow of these emotions is sinking and downwards, there may also be incontinence of sperm or premature ejaculation. Since the adrenal glands, particularly the adrenaline response, provides the energetic support for both urinary and sexual function, or response, in the male, men who don't live a balanced, well-regulated emotional life and drain their adrenal energy will also find that their sexual performance suffers.

Female Reproductive Organs: Optimal female sexual response depends on a warm feeling of emotional closeness and intimacy with her partner. If this trust and intimacy are violated, there will be emotional trauma that can adversely affect female sexual health and response. This is not an absolute, all-or-nothing matter; there are many degrees of violation, ranging from a subliminal lack of proper tact and sensitivity in the male to outright rape and physical violation. These negative experiences will traumatize the woman, to a greater or lesser degree, depending on their severity, provoking feelings of fear and anxiety which will further inhibit sexual functioning and response. This is often called frigidity, and closes down the woman's feelings and receptivity to orgasm. Many women have had to disconnect emotionally from their sexual organs and their functioning as the only way of coping with a sexual life or circumstances that are completely unsatisfying and uninspiring. Losing a pregnancy also brings an aura of great grief and sadness to the female organs, and to the woman herself; many women take a long time to heal emotionally from a miscarriage or an abortion.

Brain: The brain comes last in our discussion of the emotional life of the organs because it's often the effect of humoral and metabolic imbalances arising elsewhere in the body, which send subtle vapors up to the brain to influence its functioning. **Choleric** vapors agitate, irritate and inflame, provoking anger, rage, envy, jealousy, or irritability. Warm, moist **Sanguine** vapors can stir up feelings of wellbeing, pleasure, sensuality or even lust. **Melancholic** vapors provoke feelings of prudence, caution, pensiveness, worry and withdrawal. Cold, wet **Phlegmatic** vapors will dull or fog up the brain, producing mental lethargy and dullness, or they will cloud objective thinking with excessive sentiment and subjectivity. However, the brain is not all effect; it can also be cause, since the kinds of thoughts that it habitually thinks can have a profound impact on the heart and its Vital Spirits, and hence on the entire Vital Faculty, for better or worse. And so, we have come full circle, and again return to the heart.

Suggested Foods and New Way of Eating

I personally eat a whole cantaloupe at least 5 days per week because I absolutely love cantaloupe. I also benefit from all the vitamins and nutrients that cantaloupe provide because I eat so much of it.

This is what my body gains in health each time I eat a cantaloupe- vitamin C 78%- vitamin A 30% - potassium 12%- copper 8% -folate 8% -vitamin B6 7% -vitamin B3 7%- vitamin B1 6% -magnesium 5% -fiber 5% -
vitamin K 4%.

It is important to look at what nutrients a food supplies to our bodies. When we arm ourselves with knowledge of what foods serve a higher purpose to our body, we began the process of training our brain to think more about health than taste. I encourage all to research what you decide to put in your mouth and ultimately your body, including your pharmaceutical medications. This is your only body and you are the master of your ship so do your very best to take care of it.

List of fruits that replenish vitamins
Cantaloupe
Papaya
Mango
Peaches
Grapes with seeds
Watermelon
Citrus fruits
Cherries
Tomatoes
Avocado
Berries
Pears
Bananas
Honeydew

List of vegetables that replenish vitamins
Spinach
Kale
Green Onion
Cabbage
Chards
Asparagus
Onions
Mushrooms
Garlic
Lentils
Yams
Broccoli
Squash/Zucchini
Peppers
Lettuce
Nuts, Grains, & Seeds

Pecans
Walnuts
Brazil nuts
Almonds
Cashew
Hazel
Macadamias
Pistachio
Pine
Sunflower Seeds
Flax Seeds
Chia Seeds
Pumpkin Seeds
 GRAINS
Quinoa
Wild Rice
Oats

The Goal is to drink at least half your body weight in *ounces* of Distilled, Alkaline, or Spring per day. Avoid using bread, rice, sugar/sweetener, of ANY kind.

80% raw fruits & vegetables & 20% cooked is the diet of discipline. This way of eating will allow you to clean out your body while also losing weight. Breads, Sugars, Sweeteners, Starches, Dairy, Meat, Sodas, create dis-ease in the body and offer no substantial nutrients. All Breads, Sugars, Sweeteners, Starches, Sodas, Meats, & Dairy create an acidic environment in our bodies, and that turns into problems with our health. Most juices that sit on the shelf **are not recommended**.

Fruits work as cleansers of our body, while vegetables are the builders. I would like you to pay attention to how you feel after every meal. I would also like you to acknowledge when you are truly hungry verses when you just want to taste food. You will see that most of our eating habits come from cravings and emotional needs.

When you rise in the morning, drink 16 oz of water (you can add lemon). "We should not eat until we have had a bowel movement. Break-Fast simply means we have fasted through the night and when we eat breakfast, we are breaking our fast."~ Sunshine
Fruit should be the first meal of the day. Smoothies, Cantaloupe, Papaya, Honeydew are all filling and offer a ton of nutrients. No added sugar or sweeteners are needed in fruit smoothies. Although many health consultants approve using agave as a sweetener, I do not recommend it because it is very hard to certify its authenticity. Fruit feeds our brain the proper sugars it needs to remain alert and active.

"Break-Fast simply means we have fasted through the night and when we eat breakfast, we are breaking our fast."~ Sunshine

Detoxing & Fasting

Detoxing and fasting is so important to the body. The average American who is not practicing a vegetarian or vegan diet consumes an average of over 250 pounds of meat per year. Besides the overload of acid that is flushed into your bloodstream, the animals that you are eating were slaughtered violently, and have intense fear racing through their bloodstream at the time of death.

These animals die with high amounts of adrenaline in there body. In turn, meat eaters eat the fear, adrenaline, rage, and sadness of the animal. It is important to not only clean our bodies of the acid that we have ingested from the animal, but also to clean our body of the emotion we have taken in from their tragic death.

Becoming a vegan or vegetarian is not only a better choice for you and your health, but it is a better choice for the animals and the earth. However, just because you are vegan does not mean you are healthy. It is easy to eat lots of starches and junk food when you are a vegetarian. Pastries, french fries, vegetarian burgers, fake meats, and sugar products create an acidic environment in the body. An acidic environment in the body can create mucus. Once it creates mucus, it can also create disease.

If you are interested in detoxing, the first thing that needs to happen is to tune in to your inner voice. Our spirit quietly whispers the actions we need to take in order to enhance our overall wellbeing. This is why the cigarette smoker already knows they should stop smoking, and the alcoholic knows that they need to stop drinking. Being obedient and disciplined to spirit is a major part of detoxing.

Detoxing and fasting is ongoing in different areas of our life, and it is not something that just happens with the cessation of food. We must acknowledge the things that we are most addicted to and shed the addiction.

Things we are most addicted to:
- Television
- Food
- Gossip
- Complaining
- Drugs
- Alcohol
- Complacency
- Avoidance
- "Idea" of what love means
- Sex
- Laziness
- Control
- Fitting in
- Internet
- Human Relationships
- Worrying
- Poverty

When we decide to detox or fast from foods, we become more aware of all the toxic people and things in our life. I personally do a raw food diet anytime I feel overwhelmed with life. I have also done herbal tea concoctions and water to cleanse my blood and thoughts. When we fast, we give our organs a chance to rest and renew.

Everyone has different levels to their need of fasting and detoxing the body, so it is not a one size fit all starter pack! If you are currently taking pharmaceutical medications, you will have a different detoxing program from someone who is not taking medications. Books that only focus on detoxing have been listed in the back of this book.

We are all programmed with our own internal rebooting system, so while I must advise that you seek a health professional's guidance before taking any medical/ medicinal supplements (including pharmaceutical), I must also ask that you tune into your own inner power and be guided by your higher self toward any healing that your vessel may need. Every natural doctor or regular doctor may not have the answers you need. I personally know that one size doesn't fit all in this healing journey, and I have received information from other ND's and MD's that may heal one client, while harming another, but you as an enlightened being are tuned directly in to the guidance you need, and you have to learn to trust it.

I remember reading a story in a book written by Wayne Dyer. He spoke of a woman who had stage 5 cancer in her body, and the doctors decided that there was nothing else they could do to help her, and she should prepare here family for her next steps. She decided to not share this news with anyone, and instead she went to a cabin in the woods with no cell phones so she couldn't communicate with the outside world. After going through deep meditations and affirmations, she eventually was cleared of a cancer that the doctors had originally written a death sentence for.

Too many times, we place our faith in sources outside of ourselves and disregard our own intuition when the inner-GOD attempts to direct our path. We have the power to heal ourselves from the inside, out. These are the lessons we all must master.

"Ye are Gods, and all of you are children of the most High." ~ Psalm 82:6

Because detoxing properly is such a sensitive process, I choose not to cover it entirely, but have recommended books listed in the back that specifically focus on this subject. Detoxing can be a simple process, but it is also a serious process that requires discipline and patience with yourself. *Be patient with yourself.*.

Herbs, Fruits, Vegetables & Nuts for Ailment

AIDS Herbs-Burdock, Yellow Dock, Chapparal, Hyssop, Red Clover, Licorice
AIDS Foods- 80-100% Raw Vegan Diet

Anemia Herbs - Fo ti, Dong Quai, Devil's Claw, Alfalfa, Dandelion, Pau D'arco
Anemia Foods-Dark Leafy Vegetables, Prunes, Chickpeas, Beans, Nuts & Seeds

Arthritis Herbs- Juniper, Yucca, Burdock, Wild Yam
Devil's Claw, Black Cohosh, Alfalfa, Turmeric
Arthritis Foods- Vegan diet (No meat or dairy or foods that cause inflammation)

Asthma Herbs- Blue Cohosh, Anise, Sage, Horny Goat Weed, Mullein, Ginger
Asthma Foods- Avocado, Kale, Garlic, Bananas, cantaloupe, Vegan Diet Recommended

Allergy Herbs- Burdock Root, Nettle, Echinacea, Hyssop,Thyme
Allergy Foods- Apples, Papaya, Tomatoes, Kale, Strawberries, Vegan diet recommended

Alzheimer's Herbs-Ginkgo, Rosemary, Gotu Kola
Alzheimer's Foods- Leafy Vegetables, Berries, Olive Oil, Beets, Lentils, Raw Fruits and

Brain Herbs- Gotu Kola, Ginkgo, Hyssop
Brain Foods- Walnuts, Coconut, Avocado,
Asparagus, Berries, Grapes, Cherries, Kiwi

Breast Herbs-Red Clover, Dong Quai, Stinging
Nettle, Black Cohosh, Sage
Breast Foods- Leafy Vegetables, Berries, Peaches,
Papayas, Kiwi, Cabbage, Tumeric

Bronchitis Herbs- Mullein, Lobelia, Slippery Elm,
Holy Basil, Red Clover, Cinnamon, Peppermint,
Burdock
Bronchitis Foods- Fruits, Vegetables, Whole
Grains

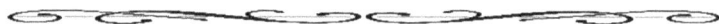

Cancer Herbs-Burdock, Yellow Dock, Red Clover,
Goldenseal, Pau D Arco, Rosemary, Prickly Ash
Cancer Foods-Vegan Raw Diet of Fruits and
vegetables recommended

Circulation Herbs-Ginger, Rosemary, Cayenne,
Blessed Thistle, Sage, Green Tea
Circulation Foods-Sunflower Seeds, Olives,
Grapefruit, Oranges, Watermelon

Cirrhosis Herbs- Gotu Kola, Milk Thistle,
Licorice, Burdock, Dandelion, Schisandra
Cirrhosis Foods-Beets, Grapes, Watermelon,
Lemon, Strawberry, Banana, Pineapple

Colon Herbs- Slippery Elm, Peppermint,
Myrrh,Black Walnut, Cascara Sagrada

Colon Foods- Bananas, Apples, Oranges, Peas, Lettuce

Common Cold Herbs- Echinacea, Ginger, Peppermint, Cayenne, Catnip
Common Cold Foods- Papaya, Grapefruit, Apples, Oranges, Peaches

Congestion Herbs- Mullein, Lobelia, Hyssop
Congestion Foods-Citrus, Berries, Tomatoes, Apples

Constipation Herbs-Cascara Sagrada, Slippery Elm, Senna, Black Walnut, Chicory, Flaxseeds,
Constipation Foods-Prunes, Figs, Apples, Kiwi, Pears, Citrus, Greens

Creatinine Levels Herbs- Ginseng, Horny Goat Weed, Horsetail, Stinging Nettle, Chamomile
Creatinine Level Foods- Pineapple, Apples, Berries, Watermelon

Depression Herbs- St John's Wort, Lotus, Lemon Balm, Rosemary, Blessed Thistle, Ginko
Depression Foods- Raw fruit And Vegetables diet

Dementia Herbs-Gingko, Gotu Kola, Bacopa
Dementia Foods- 80% Raw fruits and Vegetables and 20% cooked vegan diet recommended

Diabetes Herbs-Goldenseal, Schizandra, Burdock, Holy Basil, Turmeric, Pau D'arco, Devil's Claw

Diabetes Foods- Dark leafy greens, Beans, Berries, Tomatoes (Check potassium levels)

Diarrhea Herbs-Nettle, Corn Silk, Hawthorn, Mullein, Red Raspberry
Diarrhea Foods- Pumpkin, Bananas, Beans, White Rice

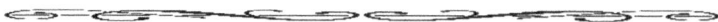

Ear Herbs- Hops, Chamomile, Lobelia, Mullein
Ear Foods- Vegan Diet Recommended

Energy Herbs- Green Tea, Astragalus, Ginseng, Oregano, Fo Ti, Schizandra
Energy Foods-Papaya, Oranges, Apples, Pineapple, Persimmons, Lemons, Dates, Peaches

Erectile Dysfunction Herbs- Tribulus, Burdock, Sarsaparilla, Horny Goat Weed, Bacopa,
Erectile Dysfunction Foods- Watermelon, Dark Chocolate, Leafy Vegetables, Nuts, Hot Peppers, Olive Oil

Eye Health Herbs- Bilberry, Slippery Elm, Eyebright, Goldenseal
Eye Health Foods- Cantaloupes, Papaya, Persimmons, Yams, Nuts

High Blood Pressure Herbs- Hawthorn Berries, Cornsilk, Holy Basil, Celery, Maringold, Cayenne, Calendula
High Blood Pressure Foods- Grapes, Berries, Pineapple, Oranges, Mangos, Seeds,

Heart Herbs- Hawthorn Berries, Cactus, Olive Leaf, Sage, Motherwart,
Heart Foods- Any Berries, Apples, Apricots, Bananas, Cantaloupe, Kiwi, Papaya, Peaches

Hemorrhoids Herbs- Dandelion, Nettle, Butcher's Broom, Witch Hazel, Butcher's Broom
Hemorrhoids Foods-Bananas, Raspberries, Pears, Apples, Barley, Peas, Lentils

Hepatitis Herbs-Blue Vervain, Milk Thistle, Sarsaparilla, Licorice
Hepatitis Foods- 80% Raw fruits & Vegetables Vegan Diet

Herpes Herbs-Olive Leaf, Red Clover, Sarsaparilla, Slippery Elm, Pau D'arco, Echinacea, Calendula
Herpes Foods- 80% Raw fruits and vegetables

Infection Herbs- Burdock, Yellow Dock, Slippery Elm, Garlic
Infection Foods- Oranges, Strawberries, Lemons, Pineapples, cabbage, Lima Beans

Insomnia Herbs- Hops, Valerian, Chamomile, Catnip, Passionflower
Insomnia Foods- Nuts, Kiwi, Cherries

Inflammation Herbs- Peppermint, Sage, Butchers Broom, Parsley
Inflammation Foods-Watermelon, Tomatoes, Berries, Oranges

Itching Herbs-Calendula, Yellow Dock, Witch Hazel
Itching Foods-Bananas, Berries, Seeds, Fresh Produce

Jaundice Herbs-Blessed Thistle, Burdock, Chicory, Yellow Dock
Jaundice Foods-Raw fruits and vegetables recommended

Joints Herbs- Mullein, Horsetail, Sarsaparilla
Joints Foods-Ginger, Grapes, Cherries, Avocado, Watermelon

Kidneys Herbs- Corn Silk, Motherswort, Horny Goat Weed, Palo Azul, Hops, Uva Ursi,
Kidneys Foods- Check with your PCD about your kidney function and levels of potassium

Laxative Herbs-Senna, Cascara Sagrada, Black Walnut Hull, Psyllium Husk, Slippery Elm

Laxative Foods- Prunes, Figs, Apples, Flaxseeds, Chia Seeds
Liver Herbs-Dandelion, Burdock, Red Clover, Wormwood, Milk Thistle, Sarsaparilla
Liver Foods-Grapefruit, Avocados, Cabbage

Lung Herbs- Pau D'arco, Mullein, Hyssop, Ginseng
Lung Foods- Ginger, Apples, Avocado, Peppers

Male Hormones Herbs- Dong Quai, Sarsaparilla, Damiana
Male Hormone Foods- Citrus Fruits, Cabbage, Garlic, Bananas, Watermelon, Grapes

Memory Herbs- Bacopa, Ginko, Gotu Kola, Blessed Thistle
Memory Foods- Walnuts, Coconut, Berries, Broccoli

Nausea Herbs- Ginger, Peppermint, Fennel
Nausea Foods- Apples, Water, Lemons, Bananas

Nerves Herbs- Valerian, Lobelia, St Johns' Wort
Nerves Foods-Dark Chocolate, Nuts, Avocado, Blueberries, Coconut

Obesity Herbs- Devil's Claw, Chickweed, Nettle, Dandelion
Obesity Foods- 80% Raw Fruits and Vegetables Diet 20% Cooked

Pain Herbs- Dong Quai, Valerian, Devil's Claw, Prickly Ash
Pain Foods- Ginger, Cherries, Red Grapes, Pineapple,

Palpitations Herbs-Hawthorn, Rosemary, Prickly Ash, Bugleweed, Motherwort
Palpitations Foods- Oranges, Bananas, Beets, Greens, Tomatoes

Palsy Herbs-Sage, Ginseng, Kava, Zinc
Palsy Foods- Pineapple, Avocados, Beets, Papaya, Figs

Pneumonia Herbs-Hyssop, Garlic, Irish Moss, Mullein, Slippery Elm
Pneumonia Foods- Citrus, Papaya, Water

Prostate Herbs- Saw Palmetto, Nettle, Hydrangea, Uva Ursi, Yucca, Red Clover, Green Tea
Prostate Foods- Tomatoes, Pomegranate, Papaya, Apricots, Guava, Brazil Nuts, Mushrooms

---

Skin Herbs- Maringold, Red Clover, Gotu Kola, Chaparral, Burdock, Yellow dock,
Skin Foods- Apples, Papayas, Apples, Kiwi, Bananas, Watermelon

Sperm Control Herbs- Fo-Ti, Horny Goat Weed, Tribulus, Saw Palmetto
Sperm Control Foods- Dark Chocolate, Watermelon, Walnuts, Pumpkin Seeds, Papaya

Stress Herbs- St. John's Wort, Melatonin, Lotus, Valerian, Schizandra
Stress Foods-Avocados, Walnuts, Blueberries, Cacao

Swelling Herbs-Uva Ursi, Mullein, Sarsaparilla, Hyssop,
Swelling Foods- Tomatoes, Olive Oil, Kale

Teeth Health Herbs-Catnip, Horsetail, Goldenseal, Prickly ash,
Teeth Health Foods-Strawberries, Celery, Apples

Testosterone Herbs-Dong Quai
Testosterone Foods- Spinach, Pumpkin Seeds, Pomegranate, Tomatoes

Thyroid Herbs- Bladderwack, Motherwort, Kelp, Irish Moss, Green Tea

Thyroid Foods- Garlic, Olive Oil, Peppers, Avocados

Tumor Herbs-Dandelion, Chickweed, Mugwort, Yellow Dock, Hyssop
Tumor Foods- Tomatoes, Apples, Pears, Onions, Garlic, Olive Oil

---

Ulcer Herbs-Fenugreek, Slippery Elm, Hops, Mullien, Sage, Pau D'arco
Ulcer Foods-Olives, Berries, Apples, Celery, Cranberries, Grapes, Bananas

Urination Herbs- Uva Ursi, Nettle, Corn Silk, Hydrangea, Juniper Berries, Hops, Fennel, Mugwort
Urination Foods-Celery, Watermelon,

Varicose Veins Herbs- Witch Hazel, Butcher's Broom, Dandelion, White Oak Bark, Gotu Kola
Varicose Vein Foods- Strawberries, Avocados, Apples, Celery

Vomiting Herbs- Spearmint, Lavender, Ginger, Slippery Elm
Vomiting Foods- Bananas, Applesauce

Warts Herbs-Mullein, Chaparral, Pau D'arco
Wart Foods- Garlic, Bananas, Figs

Pharmaceutical Medicine

Pharmaceutical medicines can deplete the body of major nutrients that are needed for proper functioning. The side effects of using certain medications can be life threatening, which is why it is so important to tell your doctor immediately when you feel some of the side effects that are listed on your medications. Also, mixing medications and not understanding the side effects of those particular drug interactions can be dangerous *and* induce new disease in the body. It is most important to acknowledge that many of medicinal herbs and pharmaceutical medications can have difficult and dangerous side effects when combined together.

Some Medications can also be horrible for people who already have labeled dis-ease in their bodies such as Diabetes, Lupus, etc. If a person is suffering from an organ stress (Kidney, Liver, Bladder, Heart) then they must be extremely careful about the extra medications they decide to take.

Pain Killers and your Kidneys
National Kidney Foundation's Top 5 Tips about
Pain Killers and Your Kidneys:

- Pain medications provide pain relief, but it's important to balance the potential benefits with the risk of side effects, such as kidney damage, fluid retention, increased blood pressure, and digestive issues.

- Many painkillers are available over-the-counter (OTC) while others require a prescription, but all pain medications carry a risk of side effects. Some examples of over-the-counter (OTC) pain medicines and corresponding brand names are aspirin (Bayer®), acetaminophen (Tylenol®), ibuprofen (Advil®, Motrin®), and naproxen (Aleve®). It's important to always read the label to see what type of medication you're taking.

- If you have decreased kidney function, certain types of pain medications such as NSAIDs (nonsteroidal anti-inflammatory drugs) are not recommended because they reduce blood flow to the kidneys.

- High doses and long-term use of painkillers may harm the kidneys, even healthy ones. Pain medications should be taken exactly as prescribed or as directed on the label, at the lowest effective dose, for the shortest period of time.

- Since most NSAIDs are referred to only by brand or generic name, as opposed to by the "NSAID" category, many people may not be aware that they are taking this type of medication, or may accidentally take more than one NSAID at a time. Approximately 23 million Americans use nonprescription (over-the-counter) NSAIDs every day.

Speak up and ask questions in your doctor's office and at the pharmacy. People with underlying kidney problems may be particularly sensitive to NSAIDs. Talking with your doctor about it can help manage concerns and prevent further damage to the kidneys.

Drugs that can contribute to liver damage

Prescription Drugs
  Antibiotics:
- Erythromycin.
- Amoxicillin-clavulanate.
- Tetracyclines (doxycycline, minocycline, tetracycline)

Antipsychotic drugs:
- Risperidone.
- Chlorpromazine.

Statins (treats high cholesterol).

Antifungal drugs:
- Terbinafine.
- Ketaconazole.

Antihypertensives:
- Lisinopril.
- Captopril.
- Methyldopa.

Halothane (anesthetic).

Antidepressants:
- Setraline.
- Fluoxetine.
- Bupropion.

Anticonvulsants:

- Phenobarbital.
- Carbamazepine.
- Phenytoin.

A Man's Cry for Health

Pharmaceutical Drugs & their Nutrient Depletion

Anti-Diabetic Drugs (ex.Metformin): Nutrients depleted- B-12, Folic Acid, CoQ10

Diuretics (ex. Furosemide) : Nutrients depleted- Magnesium, Potassium, B1, B6, C, Calcium, Potassium, Zinc, Sodium

Drugs for High Cholesterol (Statins ex. Lipitor): CoQ10, Vitamin A, A12, Vitamin D, E, Beta-Carotene, Folic Acid, Iron

Antacids (ex.Maalox/Pepcid): Vitamin B12, D, Iron, Calcium, Zinc, Folic Acid

Antibiotics (ex. Penicillin/ Augmentin): B Vitamins, Vitamin K, Beneficial Intestinal Bacteria, Calcium, Magnesium, Iron

Anti-Depressants (ex. Zoloft): B12, Folic Acid, CoQ10, Omega 3

Anti Inflammatories (ex. Cortisone): Vitamin C, D, Calcium, Magnesium, Potassium, Selenium, Folic Acid, Zinc

Beta Blockers/Hypertension (ex. Metropolol): Melatonin, CoQ10

*Antacids (ex. Pepcid):*Vitamin B12, D, Folic Acid, Zinc, Iron
Statins for Cholesterol (ex. Lipitor): CoQ10

127

Pain Medications (ex. Tylenol): Vitamin C, Folic Acid, Zinc

With all medications, both herbal and pharmaceutical, the key is to understand that both forms of medicine are not a Band-Aid. Your diet should be your primary focus for your overall health. Herbs were the first medicine of the earth, but you cannot take herbs for high cholesterol and then keep consuming your favorite fried chicken and burgers! If you truly want change in your health, you must re-learn the importance of eating foods that are medicinal and decide to make a lifestyle change.

The side effects of not being in control of your own health are life threatening, and you cannot continue to put poison in your body and expect ultimate health. Yes, pharmaceutical medication can be extremely dangerous, but the thing that is happening inside your body, which has caused you to need these medications, is the real issue.

Study your body. Study your labeled disease. Study the foods you eat and ask yourself, "Is this food helping my health, or helping me decline?" You are in control of what you decide to consume, be it burgers, pharmaceutical medications, drugs, negative energy, etc. and you have the power at any given moment to change your perspective, thus changing your reality. I love you.

A Man's Cry for Health

Interviews of Men

I have written this book as a woman who just happens to have many wonderful male friends in my life as well as clients that have openly shared their mishaps in male/Female relationships as well as physical/mental/ and spiritual health. The information provided in this book is somewhat based on what I feel is needed to help men who are on a journey to find out some of the holistic ways to care for self, but also the basic 101 education about the male body from a physical and spiritual perspective.

The reality is; I am writing this book from the divine guided assistance of the most high and other contributors. I completely understand that I am not a man, and even as the words have flowed through my vessel, I have learned the places in my own life that I must apply change because I have operated out of ignorance.

This interview section is from some of the most wonderful men I know, and they range from Shamans, to Priest and Spiritualist, Reiki Masters, Business Men, Poets, and Artist.

I asked all of these men the same questions, and they all answered in their own divine opinion. Their answers were not edited beyond needed punctuation, because I wanted to leave the rawness of their expressions available to all who read, and not alter their statements as a whole.

A Man's Cry for Health

The Questions

1. As a man, what do you wish women understood more about men?

2. When you are stressed what can a woman do to help?

3. Have you ever had Suicidal Thoughts?

4. What do you think your biggest challenges are in health as a man?

5. Who do you think is the perfect mate for you?

Rev. Shawn Wells Goldman- Founder of Spirit
Science Institute/Subtle Body Surgeon/
Metaphysician/Shaman/Astrologer/ Holistic
Practitioner/Ordained Minister
Email-shamanhandsinfo@gmail.com
Phone- (404) 709-7952 (909)705-9761

*As a man, what do you wish women understood
more about men?*

Wow. What a way to start off an interview! I feel like
I could actually write an entire book answering just
this one question! However, if I had to narrow it
down, what I would love women to understand
primarily is that men are not women. We are
different. In addition, as obvious and trivial as that
may seem, we have specific types of differences that
can cause debilitating struggle and unnecessary
challenges when we are unaware of them. Many
women (and men, for that matter) would benefit
greatly from meditating on this. Moreover, men
would most certainly appreciate women taking the
time to contemplate over the concept of our
differences and its many implications.

Perhaps the greatest example of this is the use of
language and how men and women communicate
with each other. The language men use is almost
completely different from the language women use.
Even if we are both speaking in the same "cultural"
language such as English, Spanish, French, etc.,
within these languages men and women are doing
very different things. We have different tendencies,

strengths, weaknesses and preferences. However, the more we understand how to become bilingual, or even multi-lingual in a sense, the better off we will be. Bottom line, we all use a non-native language.

Another important issue that I see creating problems for both men and women, is the very beliefs that many women have come to possess in regards to what men *want* in a woman. Now, let me be clear.. It is important that I make the distinction between wanting a *temporary connection due to an immature approach to relationships, and what men truly want from the heart*. When I say, 'what men want,' I am referring to spiritually mature men with solid integrity. Furthermore, when I say "want in a woman," I'm talking about the woman that this type of man longs for with his soul. She is his reason for enduring seemingly relentless turmoil in hopes to one day find her, and when he does she becomes his reoccurring relief. I can confidently say that a frightening majority of what I see women do in order to grab and keep a man's attention is extremely different than what we actually want. Unfortunately, many of the reasons for this phenomenon are directly associated with the mal-intentions of those who have manipulated the minds of the public through very real means of programming and psychological warfare. Lies, lies, lies. Lies to the point of disbelief, and to the extent that even men, themselves, have false beliefs about their OWN desires! Now that is twisted. Imagine that...a world where men repeatedly say to women (in every way you can think of) that we want certain things from and of her that actually, in truth, are some of the very things that repel, turn off, disgust and even sadden many men.

Confusing enough? Right, I know. But that's the nature of the programming we received. Turn us against each other and influence our behavior so that we unknowingly push each other further and further away by any means available. Therefore, we end up in a world where we automatically associate women with things like excess makeup, unnatural hair and basically anything that covers the parts of her that we are longing to see (mainly her authentic face and natural hair). Meanwhile, on the opposite end of the spectrum we are also associating women with extreme exposure of certain areas of the body that men naturally prefer to honor and respect due to the sacredness these areas represent. Again, I want to be clear. These are men with solid integrity I'm speaking of.

As confusing as our situation can become at times in the midst of figuring out how to maneuver through the uncertainties, I HIGHLY encourage women to focus less on what she has been *taught* men want, and more on learning the nature of the psychological warfare at play around her. Even what she has been taught about her own desires is false in most cases. I speak for men all over the world (even the still unawakened ones who would disagree with me) when I say, simply put, we want you. Period. The real you. No additives, no fillers, cover-ups, or camouflage. No changes to your skin, eyebrows, nails, eyelashes, breast size, or any other part of your body. Bottom line, from our perspective a woman is the most beautiful physical manifestation in all of creation. My question to women everywhere who feel the need to change their appearance for any reason at all would be, "My beloved sister, how do you correct perfection?" Wanting to change it for fun or artistic endeavors is understandable, but many of the reasons I find hiding beneath the ones that actually get expressed are associated with a strong sense of necessity, loneliness, self judgement, and a significant lack of self-acceptance. However, much is changing on our planet in regards to what is known to be true about ourselves as opposed to what is merely believed. I would say to my sisters, look toward the men you feel are true from the very core of your being. They will help you understand men. As a matter of fact, many of us would consider it an honor and a privilege to assist with such a process and drop everything we are doing in order to engage in the opportunity with pleasure!

I could go on and on, listing more and more things, but I'll end with this important one...our simplicity. Men are simple. Katt Williams said it. Sinbad said it. I'm pretty sure Dave Chappelle has said it in a number of ways as well as several other comedians. To me, it's interesting how such a seriously important truth can wind up in the presentations of so many that focus on promoting humor. Both Katt and Sinbad even go as far as to show evidence of widely felt male frustration as they give us a detailed breakdown of what exactly they mean by the "men are simple" claim. Men may watch these comedy shows in a woman's presence and laugh right along with her, but most of these same men also have in the back of their minds the hope that she didn't just laugh, but also chose to give the concept some serious consideration.

Most women would be surprised how little we want as men, and not only that but also how little we need in order to remain strong protectors and providers. Yet, much of what we actually do need tends to be difficult for women to understand, or perhaps believe. For instance, and this goes back to the communication differences, men absolutely love explicit instructions. When men say, "We don't know what you want," we truly mean it. We *want* to know, and while I acknowledge that men do need to step it up in the area of paying attention and figuring certain things out without a woman's direct guidance, it is also her responsibility to be upfront and honest with him about her truest needs. However, being upfront seems to be extremely difficult for most women due to the belief that once he knows what she needs it will scare him away, because he will not be willing or able to accept the challenge. Trust me, not knowing what a woman's individual needs are for too long due to undisclosed information will "scare him away" for sure. Tell him what it is and you will get it. Even if he is not the man to provide it for you, remain honest with both yourself and others and the man who truly is the one will show up.

When you are stressed, what can a woman do to help?

Connection through silent touch is one of the most powerful things a woman can do for a man who has made room for her in his heart. Much more than most people realize and far too often, men feel unwanted. Men do not receive loving touch nearly enough and this is already the truth even when we are babies.

When a woman reaches out to touch us we can experience unbelievable healing before the physical connection is even made. Just seeing her willingness to reach towards us can turn our entire life around in an instant and I'm not exaggerating. I cannot count the number of times in the past that I have been in an intense disagreement with a mate, angry and confused to the point of nearly paralyzed trying not to explode in rage - only to experience an unexpected shift in emotions upon noticing her gentle hand approaching mine. And as if that wasn't enough, these shifts would be followed by a sudden and unexpected emotional release with tears beginning to run down my face at the exact moment of receiving the soft, considerate touch on my hand. Once again, I learned I was wanted.

Many times when men "leave," whether it is permanent or just in order to "get some air" and calm down, they are not leaving because they truly *want* to leave. Much of the time, probably more than most people are willing to admit, they are leaving because they truly believe they are not wanted. This also goes back to the language differences and the fact that most men and women have not been taught how to read each other properly. I would say to my sisters, if you want to see some "quick fixes" when he's stressed, even if you think he's stressed because of anger towards you, then remember this - touch his hands often, rub his back often, and rub his scalp often.

Most women have no idea the power of simply placing their hands in a man's hair or on the top of his head and gently massaging his scalp or rubbing her fingers through his hair. This INSTANTLY calms a man down from ANY type of stress he is feeling. You don't need to say a word. As a matter of fact, silence specifically helps because talking and presenting him with questions will weaken him in high stress situations, especially if the questions are about his feelings. So if questions are presented, you will want to make sure they are absolutely necessary because of safety reasons. Otherwise, if he is not initiating conversation he doesn't want to talk right now. And if you offer silent compassion, genuine presence, and gentle touch all at the same time, he will feel much safer with you emotionally and perhaps even physically.

Also, giving a man space is also very necessary at specific times. This can be extremely difficult for emotionally involved women who are in many cases in need of his physical presence for comfort and a strong sense of protection in the very moments he is in need of his space. Part of this comes from her strong connection to him and his feelings, even if he is disconnected from his own emotions. Thus, when he feels off she feels off. You know the famous phrase, "If momma ain't happy, ain't nobody happy," right? Well, "momma" applies to women in general. For men, it's more like, "If poppa ain't happy, momma knows." However, even if "momma knows," more times than not she is still unclear about what exactly it is that he is unhappy about and why. Here's the added challenge - he's unclear too. And not only that but men have a very different way of gaining clarity than women do when extremely upset, especially if it involves actually being upset *with your partner.*

Women can many times figure things out by being able to have a strong sounding board that allows them to express OUT LOUD everything that they are currently feeling and thinking so that they can hear it, themselves. Once they are able to actually hear their own thoughts outside of their own mind, from their own mouth with the support of an attentive listener, clarity begins to rush in. For men, the process is very different and in many ways completely opposite.

In order for men to figure things out while upset, we absolutely NEED to think within our own minds along with the ability to focus for extended periods of time. This means without interruptions or distracting sounds (especially someone talking to us), or anything that would continue to pull us away from our thought process. When men are in the middle of processing thoughts and emotions in order to gain clarity, it takes a lot of concentration.

In recent years I was taught one of the greatest analogies I have ever come across regarding the differences in men and women - men hunt deer; women gather berries. Now stay with me... Men do not spend anywhere close to the amount of time talking as women do. This is even true for highly talkative men, such as myself. We have to know how to communicate with our brothers in silence in order to survive in many cases. Picture men out in the woods together on a very serious mission to bring back food for everyone in the village. Noise will scare the food away, but they must communicate with each other because they are a team. Men have developed a remarkable ability to engage in silent communication with one another. We use everything from hand, head and arm gestures to silent facial expressions. It takes intense concentration to do this with each other whether or not prey is even detected. However, if the prey is found, making any noise at all becomes a huge mistake. One small sound could literally be the difference between everyone in the village having something to eat and everyone going hungry.

With his bow and arrow drawn, even if he has managed to get into this position quietly, a hunter may only have one shot. He absolutely MUST take his time to "get it right," and if he misses, makes noise, or is distracted from his focus, then he will more than likely have to start all over from scratch attempting to achieve the very same thing. Now he has much less energy to accomplish his goal and probably with feelings of disappointment. Imagine the frustration that he would likely feel after using so much energy just to accomplish one main objective, and after hours and possibly even days of searching for an opportunity, it is ruined within an instant. It is important to note that the same silent approach by a man would be even more important if he is the one being hunted, himself, by an enemy who has not yet detected his location. In THIS instance, one sound or distraction could mean far worse than going hungry for a while. It could be the end of both his life and the lives of those he is protecting and providing for. The bottom line is that when stressed, whether due to extreme focus or extreme discord, men need silence and in many cases isolation, but specifically isolation from women. So, if silent scalp rubs, silent back rubs, or silent attempts to reach for his hand aren't working, he needs space. If he receives the space he needs, he will return a more capable person.

There are several scenarios of a man's "off" feelings being accompanied by a state of extreme confusion within him, which makes isolation necessary. To a woman, however, the amount of isolation time that he needs can feel like more than she can bare. Something that can help with this is a lesson I received from Mat Boggs, author of "Cracking The Man Code." I like to refer to it as the "rubber band exercise." This is for women everywhere, so share this with your sisters far and wide. As a woman, whenever you are experiencing a man pulling away from you, imagine that you are connected to him by an unbreakable rubber band. It is the elasticity of the rubber band and the force of its own pull when stretched to the limit that will bring his physical presence back to you. Therefore, if you "go after him" in an attempt to keep him from leaving you, you are actually preventing the rubber band from doing the work for you and prolonging the process. The more you keep the distance constant by moving toward him as he is moving away from you, the more he needs to move away from you even further in addition to now needing even *more* isolation time than he previously needed because now he has to also process the idea that his need for space is not being respected. But rest assured, with enough patience, trust and honoring of his needs, he will come rushing back to you. This is because you have allowed the rubber band to stretch enough to where he can no longer increase the distance between the two of you without feeling the discord that comes from remaining isolated for too long. Eventually he will not be able to stand it either.

It takes practice for men to locate the fine balance between being physically present with you and maintaining the space that they need at certain times, and that is if he is even aware of this dynamic at all because most men aren't. Yet, a simple understanding of how a woman's very presence naturally lowers a man's "feel good" chemical, dopamine, can help men and women get through these moments much easier. At least a basic understanding of this is crucial because her "feel good" chemical, oxytocin, actually increases with his presence. His, however, goes down. So argument or not, he's going to need some alone time after a while to recharge and rebuild the energy that you actually need from him.

I really could go on and on, in order to wrap up my answer - let it be known that for men, nothing compares to massage, massage, massage! Remember, touch is a major key with men. MAJOR! We are not touched enough. If it becomes a regular thing, it is healing for us in ways that I will not even attempt to describe. If you want to immediately disarm a man who is wanting to engage in conflict instead of isolating himself, begin massaging his shoulders and the muscles around his spine. It will be your own magic working before your very eyes.

Have you ever had suicidal thoughts?

Oh, absolutely! I can remember having them as a youngster in high school, and then again later in life in my mid to late twenties, especially right after my divorce. While the pain from the divorce was certainly the greatest out of all of the emotionally damaging experiences I'd ever had, I came to learn that much of my own reasons for suicidal thoughts even prior to that centered around the idea of feeling extremely lonely on this planet. It was as if I had to accept the fact that I was the only one of my kind so to speak. Soon enough, I was introduced to the concept of indigo children. That explained pretty much everything for me. I understood more and more about myself as I continued to research and explore the subject of indigo children through the work of Wan Chi Kim, Doreen Virtue, Neale Donald Walsch, and many others. But honestly, in my line of work over the years now as a shaman and metaphysician, even outside of working directly with indigos and other "starseed" children, I would be amazed and overly delighted to find even a handful of people who have NOT ever had suicidal thoughts on this planet at this time. That is, if they have at least made it to their teenage years. This is greatly due to the nature of the planet shifting into higher consciousness. In response to this shift there are those who are struggling to maintain the outdated paradigm by promoting an awareness of lack, self-judgement, and a strong sense of separation. Both loneliness and a sense of purposelessness can thrive off of this type of mental and emotional manipulation.

As a man, other triggers can accompany this feeling of purposelessness and even worthlessness when faced with the idea of living in such a world where visions of achieving practical sovereignty and having the ability to protect women and children are a struggle to even build in the imagination. For me, the divorce was one of these added triggers. That was 8 years ago, and back then I couldn't have told anyone where I would be 7 days in the future, let alone 8 years. I truly believed for a while that my life was over and I had no reason to go on. Thankfully, I came across a book on relationships called, "The Vortex" by world-renown Abraham-Hicks. Determined to pull myself back together, I literally forced myself to read at least a little bit of that book every single day once I'd gotten my hands on it. By applying what I was learning within every moment that I could remember to do so, I began to feel a shift within me. My love and appreciation for life returned. 8 years later I am a completely renewed person in ways that, at the time, I wouldn't have been able to even imagine. Reading that book saved my life.

What do you think your biggest challenges are in health as a man?

As a man, I think my biggest health challenges reside in 1) knowing what exactly the male physiology actually needs in total as opposed to the needs of the female physiology, and 2) understanding women's specific health needs, but especially concerning my role within our relationship dynamics as a source of support. This is true regardless of what the dynamics may be, whether it is my mate and divine reflection, one of my many beautiful sisters, or even mother figures. There is so much to learn about the ways in which men and women need each other. In such a pivotal period on our planet it is imperative that we continue to study, research and even question our own beliefs and previous conclusions.

It is also worth mentioning that men can very easily feel defeated by all the lies and miseducation it seems we must sift through over and over to find the truth about what our real health needs are. Men will go to war, especially for women, but we are in the midst of a *silent* war that directly influences our health every single day through the manipulation of our food, water, and the very air we breathe. Men can easily feel defeated by this when they are aware that they don't know what to do about it. This used to apply to me as well.

Who do you think is the perfect mate for you?

Oh that's easy. My perfect mate is the mate I have now. Our life together defies words. However, my serious, ultimate, "true blue" answer is my own higher self. And as corny or cliche' as that may sound, I'm taking it there because people really need to know that there is no more perfect mate than their higher self, and it is only when your relationship with self has been strengthened, cultivated and appreciated that one can even find their preferred reflection in another person. I'm honored to say that this has now been my experience. They will be different for everyone, but they will be perfect.

Any other questions or insight you would like to add, please do.

Toni (Alika), I am so grateful to have merged experiences with you in this life, and apparently other previous lifetimes. I have studied your work for quite some time now and will always remember how immediately you grabbed a space in my heart when I first met you. You were promoting your book, "Chemical Suicide" at Sevananda Natural Foods Market in Atlanta, Georgia in order to help women know the truth about certain dangers they were unknowingly exposing themselves to on a regular basis. Shocking for many of us, the dangers are in the form of poisons disguised as beauty products, hair care, hygiene essentials, etc. When I actually heard your story during the talk you gave that day, especially after your tear-filled answer to the question I asked in the audience, the part of my heart that was already yours melted completely. I believe we share a passion for helping others experience true pain relief and health recovery on a grand scale, as well as for the individual. You have touched my life in ways that words cannot capture, you are an unmeasurable inspiration, and I am honored to serve as your brother on this path of healing and teaching. I love you!

A Man's Cry for Health

Lateef McLeod- Author, Poet, Activist
www.lateefmcleod.com

*As a man what do you wish women understood
more about men?*

What I wish women understood more about men is
that it may be harder to express our feelings and
emotions, but when we share them with you it means
that you are very special in our lives.

When you are stressed what can a woman do to help?

Women can empathize with what we are going
through and be there for them and we will reciprocate
and do the same thing for them.

Have you ever had Suicidal Thoughts?

Yes, of course. Being in an ableist, racist, and
capitalist society as a black man with a disability my
identity, like many other people get negated. As a
byproduct of the oppressive hierarchical structures, I
have felt marginalized and ostracized by some
aspects of social life and thought that people will pay
attention to me more when I am dead. Also, the
devaluation of the disabled body in the current
society makes people like myself feel we would be
better off dead than alive. However, it is up to people
with disabilities to change the narrative to that story.

What do you think your biggest challenges are in health as a man?

My biggest health challenges are to have a healthy diet and have enough exercise. With health concerns like diabetes to worry about these are serious health concerns. Along with psychological stresses because I sometimes feel that I cannot express my feelings adequately and until I started seeing a psychologist I was holding a lot inside.

Who do you think is the Perfect Mate for you?

The perfect woman for me is one that will understand where I am coming from. She will share my interests and we will support each other in our endeavors. We will both have a strong spiritual grounding and a wide interest in intellectual pursuits. We will also enjoy exercising and travelling together.

___

Instructor Chris- Reiki Master, Tai Chi and Chi Kung Instructor.
Kawmefreedomspath@gmail.com
832 821 4949

What do I wish women knew about men?
That men are emotional just like women and that when a woman speaks life into a man it help him feel like he makes a difference in the world and that he is needed!

When men are stressed what can women do to help?
Be willing to listen to us and allow us to vent just like we do for you as women!

Have I ever felt suicidal?
Yes I have.

My biggest health challenge as a man is?
I feel that my biggest health challenge as a man is excepting the change that comes with getting older and making sure that we get our regular check ups that we need to have yearly!

What and who is the perfect mate for me?
The perfect mate for me is someone who keeps it 100!
A woman that know how to cook!
A woman who believes in team work
A curvaceous woman
A woman that is balanced in her thinking and emotions

A woman that wants to build an empire with me that
will turn into a legacy
A spiritual woman(God) in all things
A romantic and sensual woman
A women that wants children
A woman who will speak life into my spirit when I
am feeling low and when I feel like I can't make it!
A drama free woman!

Dr.Congo- Unorthodox Priest, Artist, Alchemist.
For readings or spiritual jewelry, contact Dr. Congo
at *dr.congo8@yahoo.com*

*As a man what do you wish women understood more
about men?*

I wish, that women understood that men have a heart
with feelings and emotions as well, but we may have
a different way of conveying what we may be going
through. Also, never take for granted when a man is
trying to express himself, even if you think that he
should do it with a certain amount of passion.

*When you are stressed what can a woman do to
help?*

In most cases just don't push a (man) and ask to many
questions at that time. If you see that he is not ready
to discuss the matter, give him time because
eventually he will talk about it especially if it is about
the relationship.

Have you ever had Suicidal Thoughts?

Yes I have had suicidal thoughts. Spirit has protected me each time I put the gun up to my head and pulled the trigger, which is a big reason I have invested a lot of time in helping others who may be leaning toward similar thoughts. As a spiritualist and a unorthodox priest, it is my responsibility to help others because of my promises to spirit(s).

What do you think your biggest challenges are in health as a man?

Eating healthy on a regular basis.

Who do you think is the Perfect Mate for you?

A woman with some similarities, but not the same. Spiritually, and on a mundane level she brings some type of balance to me as I would her.

A Man's Cry for Health

Chad Joseph (Business Man)

As a man what do you wish women understood more about men?

As a man I wish women understood more that men are victimized and divided by the same system that holds them back. Instead of supporting one another, we've been convinced that competing against each other and bashing each other is more important than nation building. We've suffered the same traumas and chose to compare our scars vs healing one another.

When you are stressed what can a woman do to help?

When a man is stressed I think the best thing a woman can do is be a good listener. Women are the best problem solvers because they first listen to each other, separate the emotion, and filter down to the facts. Men are so solution based that they don't realize how valuable this process is. We are taught to pay for a solution or solve it physically (go see an expert, work harder, etc) when the proven way for thousands of years is: verbalize the problem to an understanding person and find the solution within.

Have you ever had suicidal thoughts?

I've never had suicidal thoughts but I can understand the (false) concept of dying to end suffering. Growing up as capitalists, we have watched human life become a commodity. We don't value it as much as we should. People are ready to die for the flag, die for hiphop, die for their jewelry. People wanting to die to end suffering is a natural result of that.

What are your biggest health challenges as a man?

 As a man our biggest health challenges are diet and stress. I think both lead to 99% of our problems.

Who do you think is the Perfect Mate for you?

The perfect mate for me shares my goals, understands my challenges, is motivational, and loves being pampered.

Marrio Marshall-
Studio Owner, Music Production, Music Editing,
Video Editing, Graphics.
678-886-1780
www.mlmediallc.com

As a man what do you wish women understood more about men?

I don't like the wishy washy indecisiveness. In my opinion, a woman shouldn't ask questions they already know the answer to. Be honest and be able to take everything you decide to dish out. I believe a woman should know her role. If you expect me to take out the trash and be the man of the house, I expect you to play your part and not try to infringe on my role.

When you are stressed what can a woman do to help?

The best thing a woman can do for me is be quiet and give me space. She must understand that everything isn't always about her all the time and men actually have feelings too. We are not robots.

Have you ever had suicidal thoughts?

Yes I have. I think lots of people have dealt with similar issues. Life is hard, and for some people life can be a true burden. People will attempt to eliminate their pain by completely erasing themselves from the equation. Some people are depressed, some are just tired of life's pain and just want to get out of the cycle completely.

Many times those who want to commit suicide chase a high that they will never reach again. It's almost like a constant failure that you endure over and over. People that want to commit suicide most of the time are creative in nature, but it's a constant void that they can never fill because being creative is like a high. Unfortunately, when these creative people reach their highest point it's hard to go backwards from there.

What are your biggest health challenges as a man?
Eating right and dealing with the psychological stresses that society has placed on us as men.

Who do you think is the Perfect Mate for you?
There is no such thing as a perfect mate in my opinion. At the end of the day it just depends on what you are willing to deal with. It is like you have to ask yourself, "Do I like this woman enough to deal with her hang ups and vice versa," because we all have them.

Last words..
If a man was not shit when you met him, most likely he won't be shit later on. Men are not Ken dolls, so stop trying to make men what you want them to be and either accept them for who they are or move on to the next.

A Man's Cry for Health

A message from Toni *and* Spirit

I believe, like all other disease, Dementia is caused by having too much mucus on the brain. I also believe that if the diet is reversed and patient is placed on a raw fruit and vegetable juice diet, the brain will slowly be cleared of excess mucus and dementia will eventually disappear.

I believe most disease is caused by the choices of foods we decide to put in our mouth, *as well as* the choices of emotions we choose to hold in our soul. The bad choices in foods create toxin build-ups & promote excess mucus in our bodies and around our organs, thus causing disease. In addition, holding on to negative emotions can cause stagnation in our energy force and interrupt the release of necessary energy to heal.

I have learned that men who are stuck on a superficial level of *a*wareness are more concerned with a woman being arm candy verses brain food.

Self-correction is mandatory for positive elevation. We must constantly be able to acknowledge the faults of our own, but also acknowledge our ego when it tries to *convince* us to choose destructive habits through false negotiation with our higher self.

The brain is an amazing organ, and if we truly want to heal our life, the brain will produce the healing blueprint for the body. Our duty is to be obedient to following the blueprint that GOD provides.

When you tell a cigarette smoker that they need to stop smoking, the cigarette smoker will tell you all the compromises they have made as a response from their *lower self,* to keep the habitual agreements of knowingly causing harm to the body. This same concept applies to all the different ways we cause harm to others and ourselves. We have compromised with our lower self and willingly gone against our higher being in order to remain at a lower frequency.

80%- 100%-raw fruits and vegetables, and 20% cooked is the diet of a healing body.

A happy penis is Hap-pi-ness!

Some of the foods that create mucus are- Sugar, Meat, Dairy, Processed foods, Yogurt, Soy, Eggs, Butter, Bread, Starches, Alcohol. If you want to heal the body, the first step should be eliminating the foods that cause excess mucus.

I believe depression comes when we have not learned to master our thoughts. It is so easy to imagine the worst-case scenario, and then act out on what we imagine through the emotion our imagination has inspired. We must train the brain to imagine greater outcomes for ourselves, We must also understand that our feelings of depression shouldn't be permanent. One of the most valuable lessons I learned in my holistic health class was, "The only healthy emotion is peace."

Inspirational Quotes

It's not the load that breaks you down, it's the way you carry it. – Lena Horne

I really don't think life is about the I-could-have-beens. Life is only about the I-tried-to-do. I don't mind the failure but I can't imagine that I'd forgive myself if I didn't try. – Nikki Giovanni

If you're walking down the right path and you're willing to keep walking, eventually you'll make progress. – Barack Obama

Whatever is bringing you down, get rid of it. Because you'll find that when you're free . . . your true self comes out. – Tina Turner

In a world filled with hate, we must still dare to hope. In a world filled with anger, we must still dare to comfort. In a world filled with despair, we must still dare to dream. And in a world filled with distrust, we must still dare to believe. – Michael Jackson

You're not obligated to win. You're obligated to keep trying to do the best you can every day. – Marian Wright Edelman

If you don't like something, change it. If you can't change it, change your attitude. – Maya Angelou

Yes we can! – Barack Obama

*Find the good. It's all around you. Find it,
showcase it and you'll start believing in it.*
— Jesse Owens

What you're thinking is what you're becoming.
— Muhammad Ali

*You are no better than anyone else, and no one is
better than you.*
— Katherine Johnson

I got my start by giving myself a start.
— Madame CJ Walker

*I prayed for twenty years but received no answer
until I prayed with my legs.*
— Frederick Douglass

*Everything will change. The only question is
growing up or decaying.*
— Nikki Giovanni

*What's the world for if you can't make it up the way
you want it?*
— Toni Morrison

*If you are fortunate to have opportunity, it is your
duty to make sure other people have those
opportunities as well.*
— Kamala Harris

Recommended Reading

Relationships & Sexual Health
Holistic Sexuality by Dr. Akua Gray
The Spirit of Intimacy by Sobonfu Some
Attached by Amir Levine
She Comes First by Ian Kerner
Introduction to Tantra by Lama Thubten Yeshe and
Jonathan Landaw

Positive Thinking
Today Wellness Manifestations by K. Akua Gray
As a Man Thinketh by James Allen
The Alchemist by Paulo Coelho
Breaking the Habit of Being Yourself by Dr. Joe
Despenza
A Return to Love by Marianne Williamson
The Vortex by Abraham Hicks

Detoxing
Detox Therapy by Dr. Akua Gray
21 Day Sugar Detox by Diane Sanfilippo
Raw Food Detox by Natalia Rose
The Detox Miracle Sourcebook by Robert Morse N.D

Other Recommended Books
Hands of Light by Barbara Ann Brennan
101 Things I Wish My Father Taught Me by Jasiri Basel
Sacred Contracts by Caroline Myss
African Holistic Health by Dr. Llaila O. Africa
Back to Eden by Jethro Kloss
300 Herbs by Mathew Alfs
The Book of Secrets by Deepak Chopra

Credits: U.S. Commerce Department figures compiled for the National Confectioners Association (NCA) and the Chocolate Manufacturers Association. (Reuters, 8/21/98) (2) Beatrice Trum Humter, The Sugar Trap & How to Avoid It, (Houghton Mifflin Co., 1982), p.15. (3) Nancy Appleton, Ph.D., Lick The Sugar Habit, (Warner Books, N.Y., 1985) pp. 73,74. .

CriticExtreme-My Blog, My observations, My Truth

Dr. David Reuben- , author of Everything You Always Wanted to Know About Nutrition

National Institute of Diabetes and Digestive and Kidney Diseases

Addiction Center

National Institute of Mental Health NIMH

Cancer.org

Cancer.net

BeatCancer.org

Dictionary of Cancer

Back To Eden- Jethro Closs

300 Herbs: Their Indications & Contraindicatiions- Mathew Alfs

Natural Health & Wellness Consultant Certification Manual-Dr. K. Akua Gray ND

Men's Health

GreekMedicine.net

Wikipedia

National Institute of Health

The American Cancer Society

The American Heart Association

The American Kidney Association

The American Liver Association

DrugAbuse.com

Diabetes & Sexual & Urologic Problems NIDDK

AddictionCenter.com

Thank You, Toni

Follow on all social media at
@therealtonihickman